The
Heart of
Happiness

Restoring Happiness
with Heart-Centred Healing

Julienne Rose

BALBOA
PRESS

A DIVISION OF HAY HOUSE

Balboa Press books may be ordered through booksellers or by contacting:

Balboa Press
A Division of Hay House
1663 Liberty Drive
Bloomington, IN 47403
www.balboapress.com.au
1-(877) 407-4847

ISBN: 978-1-4525-1098-9 (sc)
ISBN: 978-1-4525-1099-6 (e)

Printed in the United States of America

Balboa Press rev. date: 10/10/2013

Table of Contents

Acknowledgements

I've often read this section in books and thought them to be a bit corny but now I finally get it. When you're putting your heart down on paper, in this case literally, having positive support can make all the difference. Firstly, I give gratitude to my mother and sister, for taking the time to help edit my book and not being offended in any way by the sometimes personal content of my disclosures.

Also, to the two beautiful souls who contributed their artistic gifts in the form of the beautiful book cover art work by my friend Sonja Rusden, and the poem by Olivia Cooper.

Thank you to Rob Williams, the founder of PSYCH-K. I am one of his Community of Instructors and his genuine dedication has inspired me to pursue my own path.

And finally, my love and gratitude to my two children, Jessica and Daniel, who have been my greatest teachers in the art of unconditional love.

Hearts Genius . . .

We all have our own genius
Look inside the heart
Love the heart enough to foster what is truly there
From here all clarity as to what that genius is becomes apparent
And everything in life makes sense
And we just know what blessings are here now and what blessings come next
This is our genius
Our truest nature
So
Learn to listen
Deeply listen
And be willing to understand
And live from this place
This is our true life's path
and where we truly come to know peace
For this is our true home
the home of our soul
where the most nurturing of growth healing and wisdom unfolds . . .
Enjoy the journey
And the warmth that grows every moment within this eternally loving
heart of yours
For your very own spiritual home is always with you
here now and forever

By Olivia Cooper

Principles of Heart Happiness

♥ Heart Happiness comes from your heart not from your head.

♥ Heart Happiness is a natural state of being that everyone holds.

♥ Heart Happiness can transform any area of your life.

♥ Heart Happiness comes from within you, not externally.

♥ Heart Happiness extends from every cell in your body to every part of the Universe.

♥ Heart Happiness is something we all have the ability and right to achieve.

♥ Heart Happiness transforms and transcends all other states of being.

Introduction

If we really love ourselves, everything in our life works.

Louise Hay

*I*magine being able to go beyond the limitations of the mind and directly access your Higher Self to help you with the challenges in your life? To my surprise, that is exactly what I experienced in early May 2012, when I received Higher Self guidance, firstly for myself, and then to share this information with others through **The Heart of Happiness**.

This was also at the time of the Wesak Moon, Buddha's birthday, when many people around the world received intuitive downloads. I was fortunate to be open to receiving this information in the form of messages and meditations.

The purpose of **The Heart of Happiness** is to restore happiness in people's lives with a simple process of heart-centred healing.

The Heart of Happiness is a multi-dimensional perspective, between human and spirit around seven major issues of Life; Self, relationships, health and wellbeing, career or calling, abundance, connecting with others, and love and healing.

Each chapter firstly shares my human experience, which provides the platform for the following spiritual guidance, through the messages and meditations. In sharing these experiences, I hope the reader will gain insights and parallels to assist in their own lives.

Interactive in style, this book is designed not just to be read but to be integrated into daily life through the daily practice of being in the heart space.

I never planned on writing a book as that has never been one of my ambitions in life. It came as a complete surprise to me, when along with the other material in the spiritual download, I received the guidance to put it all into a book. The messages and meditations were the easy part as all I had to do was transcribe what I had been given.

The other aspect, my human experience, has been quite a different story, literally. I listen to the messages and meditations many times and continue to do so. Even as I have been writing this book, there have been many new developments and changes in my life. Change is constant and as I receive the messages and guidance, my life transforms in new and positive ways as I hope it will in yours also.

The messages and meditations are also available in audio form on the accompanying website, www.hearthappiness.org and are free to download. At the rear of this book is a summary of meditations with a shortened, simplified version of each meditation to use on a daily basis or as needed.

About Happiness

*Happiness is not in our circumstance but in ourselves. It is not something
we see, like a rainbow, or feel, like the heat of a fire.
Happiness is something we are.*

–John B. Sheerin

What is Heart Happiness?

*H*eart Happiness is being happy. Being happy as our natural state of Being.

We often measure our head happiness by what is happening in our life right now. Yet these are external happenings. It is up to us to decide whether or not we allow them to affect our natural state of happiness.

Watch a child at play or an animal moving in nature. They are fully content and happy in the moment. What a wonderful state to be in, rather than in our head, worrying and fretting about what has gone or what might happen.

Reading or listening to the simple messages and meditations described in this book, shifts us from a state of continuously wanting and striving towards goals that seldom bring us the happiness we think they will, to a state of being happy, regardless of what is happening in our life.

Happiness is not something we have to learn or work hard at. It is our natural state of being. To remember and restore that happiness is the only task at hand. Happiness is within us at all times. If it wasn't there we would not be able to function or be alive.

To restore happiness we have to remember ourselves as we were before life's experiences added all the overlays. When we connect to our heart centre and bypass our mind, where all the overlays reside, then it is a direct channel to our happiness within. We never again need external resources, i.e. people, things, events, experiences etc, to be happy.

Human experiences are perceived uniquely, and that is all each of us has, as there is no reality, apart from our own. It took me a while to get that. It was a great shock when I finally realised that not everyone saw the world as I did. Maybe that was why there was such a feeling of disconnection and mis-communications in my life. To take that even further, I came to understand that the world I lived in and experienced was my own creation and summation of my life experiences. To be able to re-create my world and reality has been the most significant gift to myself and, in doing this, a gift also to others.

I feel very grateful and blessed to have been given the insights and understandings, through the following messages and meditations. They have helped me hugely in my personal journey dealing with my own personal challenges. I hope they help others in whatever way they are meant to.

Message: Heart Happiness

We are happiness. We are pure happiness.

Everything else around us is made up of overlays, overlays of experience, overlays of thoughts, overlays of things. Underneath all of those overlays we just are pure happiness.

From conception, even preconception, we start to accumulate these overlays that block out that light, that happiness that is always there. However, as we remove the overlays of life, we experience more and more of this pure happiness, that leads us to inner joy, and inner peace. This is what most people are seeking, as they add more and more overlays to try and find that happiness, but only become further from it.

We don't have to find happiness. Happiness is already there. We have to remember it and restore happiness. There is no point in replacing one overlay with another overlay because it is still clouding out that light. We experience moments that are close to happiness and this is what keeps us seeking it.

Undoubtedly, everyone on this planet, if we look at our behaviours and what we're doing with our lives, is in the pursuit of happiness. The irony here is, of course, that the happiness is there within us. We just have to remember it.

Where does our happiness reside? It's in all our cells and we can restore and remember our happiness through our heart. Our heart has more cells and more strength than any other organ in our body. Moving to our heart, to find that happiness, is all we have to do.

We don't have to give up all those things, experiences and people that we think have made us happy. That's all part of happiness, at least, our expressions of our happiness. As long as they are expressions of our happiness and our inner happiness is still intact, then if those things, people, experiences and objects disappear, we still have the core of happiness within us. It's not going to be upset and overturned by those changes called life.

Chapter 1
Self

Happiness depends upon ourselves.

–Aristotle

My Human Experience

*I*sn't it funny how you can go through life, and when you take the time to look back, you realize how incredibly dysfunctional your life has been? I always find it amazing how we get through and survive everything while seeming comparatively normal to the outside world.

I work with people to help them sort out their lives. Funny that, as I'm still trying to sort out my own life. Maybe they sense that my life hasn't been such a bed of roses, and it heartens them to have someone who understands life's challenges and has managed to move through them to the other side. Either way, I love what I do, and if having had a right royal screw-up of a life helps the people I work with, then that's okay.

This started out as two books and true to form, why not write two at the same time? My sister and I laugh often. We say, we're the opposite polarities of a manic/depressive. I'm the manic, and she's the depressive. We're both seeking the balance point in the middle, and now that we're both in our fifties, we're getting closer. I guess half a century is better than not at all.

I ponder on life a lot, what has happened, what is happening now, what might happen? I didn't used to get a lot of answers. I received the occasional insights, which of course didn't change things a lot, but gave me some clarity. I had lots of theories, probably most of them delusional, but fun to throw around for discussion. That is if you can find someone happy to play the game. My counselling tutor told me I was opinionated, and he was right. I love having an opinion, but I'm not too attached to it, which I think is the key. That makes me feel better about it anyway.

Life is a funny kettle of fish. When you look back at all its happenings and wonder at the busy lives we lead when we really are all preparing to die, you wonder at the seriousness of it all and why we all aren't living it up. Well, I guess some people are, but the people in my world are pretty serious. I love *'Tuesdays with Morrie'*, by Mitch Albom, with the story about the student spending time with his dying professor, saying "It's not how you die, it's how you live". So true.

As a kid, I was called selfish quite a bit as I liked to do my own thing and please myself and I still do. I love to get on with what lights me up and makes me happy. There have been a few times in my life when I've forgotten that and then I'm not a happy camper. It seems to me we get labelled in one of two ways early on, with neither label particularly useful for later life: The people pleasers and the self pleasers. We then have to find that place in the middle where our happiness allows us to share happiness and receive it without feeling guilty. I guess I'm in the latter category and because of that I can now help others as I am mostly happy with my life.

I've observed the people pleasers, and while they may make other people happy, their own lives can often be bathed in shades of grey. I wish they'd dig deep and find out what makes them happy themselves and feel okay about that. Making an art form of either extreme is where it becomes a problem and ideally I guess we try to be a bit of both and find that balance in the middle. Then, of course, there are the narcissists, and that's another whole book waiting to be written.

It's a curious thing, when you look back over your life how you only remember certain things. Scientists have explained all that through studies showing that the emotions fire the neural pathways into our minds. My memories are as insignificant as most people's. I recall as a pre-schooler, helping my mum make the beds after my older brother and sister had gone to school, feeling the satisfaction of being with her on my own. I have another memory of sitting with the local kids in the long grass at the end of the street, hearing my father yelling at my mum. I thought at first he was laughing, as he had such a loud voice. Then I realised he wasn't, and I walked home with trepidation, unknowingly having this experience set up fear in how I later interacted with the men in my life.

I remember getting my first doll and comparing my brown-haired one with my sister's blonde-haired one and realising that we were different. Mum going out at night leaving us kids on our own to catch Dad with his girlfriend. I recall seeing Dad crying, because he was leaving us, yet still not coming back, even though we all missed him so much. There were so many paradoxes.

Welcome to the world of adults and their dramas. Seemingly normal and insignificant at the time, the associated emotions attached to that experience, burned those neural pathways through my mind to rear their ugly little heads when I later ventured forth into the world of life and relationships as a teenager and adult. I went on to marry a man just like my dad; charismatic, charming and a rogue (sorry Dad). It is only recently that I have been able to connect more fully with my emotions, as this early emotional trauma of seeing my father leave in tears, made it very difficult for me to be around other people's pain, including my own. I would go to incredible lengths to avoid ending relationships, staying well over the 'best used by' date to avoid the anxiety of seeing them hurt, disregarding my own wellbeing in the process. These early painful experiences have many layers of coping and control mechanisms over them to avoid experiencing this emotional pain. Being able to go into my heart space to help me feel the emotion safely, has been a simple yet profound way of processing my emotions. I am hopeful now that I will be able to move smoothly through my daily interactions with people and loved ones, safely acknowledging and releasing emotions as they occur.

My kids have also had to deal with similar issues I had from my childhood. That's not an easy one to witness and feel okay with yourself about. I guess that's one of life's big lessons, forgiving yourself and others. It's easier said than done, as there are so many aspects of forgiveness and you can't shortcut their lessons for them by feeling guilty and rescuing them.

Having lived without much contact with my father, I was determined to give my kids a full time dad, not realising that bringing them up in a volatile environment, I was sending a message to my kids that I didn't deserve respect. They each went on in turn to treat me as he did and I was a great victim, allowing it for years. My life is very different now as I have clear boundaries and a strong sense of self worth. But it has taken me years of tough love and self-development to get there, and I'm still learning ways of coping with their behaviour whilst maintaining my love for them. Working through the layers of forgiveness, towards myself and others, takes some time and awareness. However, I do know one thing for sure, it's one of the keys to emotional freedom, peace, and happiness. I like the Buddhist philosophy, that there is no need for forgiveness if there is no blame. I now aspire to that in my life and conserve my energy for more positive things.

So who do I know my Self to be? This is a great question presented by Dzar. Dzar refers to the group of energies uniting Human and Spirit, as channelled by Mary and Gary O'Brien. Details are in the Resources Section at the rear of this book.

From what you've gleaned above, mostly I have identified with my experiences, understanding that they have shaped my sense of Self. More and more now, though, I am getting the insights and understandings that in fact none of this has much to do with anything, only if I allow it to. When I'm part way through telling my story of woe, I now catch myself and make the choice to tell it a little differently each time, with less of the pathos and victimhood. With this new understanding, I am able to be more of who I really am and less a product of my history and experiences. As I continue my spiritual path, I look forward to being more of who I truly am.

Message: Self

Connection to Self is our natural state of being. This connection to Self keeps us connected to happiness and peace within. A connection to Self is a direct line to all the wisdom and knowledge in the universe. In having this connection to Self, we have all the internal resources we need to equip us through this journey called life.

From an early age, we are taught about the Self. But unfortunately, often not in the way that would keep us connected to the Self, such as we are when we are born. We learn the words relating to self such as *self-ish, self-centred, self-less* etc. As you can see, these words have a less than desirable connotation and meaning attached to them. Knowing now that connection to Self is the most important life force for us, these words used in conjunction with our behaviour, are in fact taking us away from our true connection to Self. The irony or paradox is that the harder we try to be less of all those undesirable things, the more disconnected we become from Self.

If we realised that we already have this connection to Self, there would be no need to instruct our young ones on how to achieve this. In fact, the teachings are but social overlays of convention, apparently to give us the social skills to be accepted in our society. The cost of losing the connection to Self is too great, and many people spend their whole lives suffering due to this disconnection.

You may wonder how the child will learn to give. Yet this giving, true unconditional giving can only come from a place where there is a connection to Self in place. The most beautiful gift is from a child who gives of his or her own free will, without being prompted or cajoled. In receiving this gift of giving, we receive it in a way that is completely different than if it is given from a place of pressure.

Meditation: Establishing a Heart Connection with Self

- ♥ With eyes opened or closed, bring your attention to your breathing.
- ♥ Focus your breathing into your heart centre around the chest area and expand and energise that area.
- ♥ Know that this heart centre is the channel to your Higher Self.
- ♥ When in connection with your heart centre, your mind is still and at peace.
- ♥ If you choose to, allow a colour to fill your heart centre.
- ♥ This colour may be used to enhance and heal whatever needs to be healed.
- ♥ Know that at any time you focus your breath into your heart centre you are connected to your highest state of Being.
- ♥ The more you practice this, the more you will be free of your mind and be at peace.

Message: Soul Happiness

Our soul is the essence of us. It's the thread that runs through from lifetime to lifetime. It has no beginning, it has no end, it just is. When we connect back to our soul from our human experience, it's like returning home and being back within the core of our essence. When we have a soul disconnect, our life is fragmented and full of disturbances and difficulties. Sometimes we bring in these difficulties and disturbances from previous lifetimes, and they compound that feeling of disconnection from our soul, our soul existence, and essence. Again, these are just overlays, the residual overlays from experiences, but if not cleared and dissolved, these can have a detrimental effect on our current lifetime. To be in connection with our soul is to know true love, true love for our Self. In doing that, and having that, we then have true love for others, at the deepest level of our being.

If you look at the hug, we all use a hug to connect with others. When we hug, our heart centre, which is the seat of our soul, does a connect-up. We don't know why when we have a hug, or give a hug, or receive a hug, we feel better. It's when two souls connect. So how do we re-connect with our soul? How to re-centre ourselves back in this current lifetime, not to be confused with previous lifetimes?

For us to connect with our soul, which is within us at all times, in all lifetimes, at all levels of being, we simply need to connect to our Inner Self which is in our heart centre. When we are in this state of being heart centred, whatever goes on around us, whatever chaos, whatever experiences outside of us, and even in our own life, if we stay in that sense of soul centeredness those experiences and that chaos and that experience called life, and everything that goes with it, will just be on the periphery. We will still be able to retain our sense of Self, regardless of what other people are doing, what life situations are happening around us and in our own lives. In having that sense of Self and centeredness, we are able to access that happiness and that peace within us, regardless of anything that is happening around us, because we are that peace and happiness.

Sometimes we forget that we have the ability to do this, and yet everyone has this and everyone is this. It's not for a chosen few, and not for those who have to work hard. This is a natural state of being. It's there at all times in everyone.

Meditation: Soul Happiness

To connect to sense of Self, to that soul centre, we bring our attention to our breathing, which is our life force. Our breathing is what keeps us in this current lifetime. Without the breath we do not have life, and the breath is the channel towards this inner peace, this inner soul and inner happiness. We continue to bring our attention to our breathing, being aware of how it rises and falls, bringing that life force energy into our Being. As we bring our attention of our breathing to our heart centre, allow this to deepen and expand our chest and our breath. Each time, bring that life force energy into our heart centre, into our soul centre.

As you create this focus, notice that any current situations and events that may be happening in this lifetime. As you breath, breathing them into your heart centre and then breathing them out, allowing them to flow in and then to be released with each breath out. To support this flow and ebb, you may notice that there's a colour that comes in with each of these experiences in this lifetime. Know that these experiences that you're having in this lifetime, may in fact be a summation of all your lifetimes, or some of your lifetimes or even just one of your lifetimes.

Bring each of these experiences, that you no longer choose to have power over you in this lifetime, whether it be a person, a situation, an emotion, a state of mind, into that heart centre to be released.

Now create a heart shape in your heart centre, filling it with a colour, whichever colour you choose for this experience. To ensure that your new state of being within your heart centre and your soul is transferring to your daily thoughts, actions, behaviours and feelings, create a rainbow all the way from your heart centre up to your head. Take with it a copy of that heart, filled with that beautiful colour that you chose, and when it arrives at your head, click it into place. Click!

As we know our heart and our head are connected to that inner soul; our inner state of being, our inner Self, and that this is within us at all times, in all situations in this lifetime. When you're ready, gently open your eyes, and come back into the room.

Chapter 2
Relationships

When one door of happiness closes, another opens;
but often we look so long at the closed door that we do not see
the one which has been opened for us.

–Helen Keller

My Human Experience

When it comes to relationships, I could write a book on all my 'stuff ups' so luckily for you, you'll be getting the reader's digest version. As we are conditioned at an early age to accept what is 'normal' in the environment we're born into, I had some pretty dysfunctional ideas about what was okay in a relationship. Poor old Mum had struggled through after Dad left her for a much younger version, and through all her venting and rage, I figured out that men were pretty much redundant and useless, not to mention being completely untrustworthy. This was reinforced by only seeing Dad a couple of times a year when he'd lavish us with presents and a ride out in his yacht, or something equally extravagant, while Mum struggled to pay the bills and feed us.

So with all that software in place in my subconscious mind, including the beliefs that men were unreliable, selfish and treacherous,

9

blah, blah, blah, I embarked on a career of attracting men who were just like that, further confirming my theories (and Mum's of course).

If I'm being really honest though, my first boyfriend at age 14 was a real sweetie, so nice but SO BORING! He actually wasn't of course, but it was out of my comfort zone to have peace and calm in my life, and to be treated well by a male. I was much more comfortable with chaos, all of this at a subconscious level of course. That then led me to believe that all nice men were boring and all interesting men were bastards. You can see how they just couldn't win. After many years of failed relationships, I one day realised I had a two year pattern, where once the oxytocin, like a honey moon hormone, had worn off in my brain, off I'd go and this was a great way of ensuring I never got hurt.

It's all very well when you discover a pattern you've been running, but it would be equally great if you could then change it. Often, though, it's not that easy. My subsequent study and knowledge of how the subconscious mind operates has allowed me to do that to some degree, but prior to that it took much trial and error. One of my previous attempts led me to run an experiment where I did internet dating for three months to break my habit of being drawn to the 'wrong type'.

I had lots of fun and many forays into the dangerous and unknown, so I'm not so sure I'd recommend it, or whether it worked. I did get quite good at saying no though, so that was quite an achievement for me. I also became very good at recognising my 'moth to the flame' habit, and found it easier to make a conscious choice when I had to, rather than falling back into old habits.

I finally gave up the pattern of trying to fix the 'broken' man. I realise now that firstly he wasn't broken, just different from me, and secondly he didn't want to be fixed as things were working out very fine for him, thank you! I am now much clearer about what I want in a relationship and for now, am very happy living on my own. It feels like a great space to be in as I am free to travel and do what I please. I remember when I was younger, and when I would see an older lady on her own, I felt really sorry for her. Now I understand that in fact it is great to be on your own, and when and if you do meet that person who lights you up in a special way, then that's a bonus.

Anyway, I've made my peace with men, well most of them anyway, and actually quite like them now. I've finally learned that when you break up, you can still be friends with them. Also, that it's okay to leave a relationship if it isn't what you want, rather than vilifying them to justify your exit. I've learned something about myself from each of my relationships. In the past, my neediness was contradicted by pushing them away if they came too close. I have seen this pattern in many people around me. The wounded child cannot bear to lose them or conversely get too close, so there are no winners here. I am thankful I have left that pattern behind as it is one of the hardest to break.

My advice to people who recognise this pattern in themselves, is to do the work with yourself so you are strong and never lose that, so no matter what the outcome of the relationship is with that person, you will always have yourself intact, not broken.

As you will read in the following chapter, this good advice of mine was put to the test very recently. While I have been living on my own, I have kept one foot in a relationship, and even with this distance, I found it very challenging when faced with deception and betrayal. I finally managed to get through it by allowing myself to feel all the emotions, moving through them many times until I managed to find some peace within myself.

It finally made sense why all the messages had come through as they did, almost in preparation for what was going to happen. In allowing myself the space, I finally received even more clarity that it was not my job to 'fix' the relationship. My only responsibility was to heal myself and move towards happiness.

Message: Relationships

The relationships that we have with other people, are a direct reflection of the relationship that we have with our Self. When we heal our relationship with our Self at all levels of being, for all things, then the relationships around us have the opportunity to heal as well. This relationship with our Self includes forgiveness.

Firstly, maybe loving ourselves exactly as we are, including our physical Self, our behavioural Self, how we behave, our spiritual and emotional Self. As we love our Self for everything, this doesn't mean to say we can't make changes to our Self at some later stage, but we first need to come to a place of full acceptance of our Self.

This full acceptance of our Self then leads into acceptance of others, taking away the judgement, and the emotional reactions to what others may be doing in their lives. When we do this, we cease to be affected and buffeted around in the breeze by other people. We retain our sense of wholeness within our Self. All the relationships in our life with our family, our parents, our children, our siblings, grandparents, grandchildren, our friends, colleagues, all receive the benefit when we have this strong, solid, unconditional relationship with our Self. It gives others a sense of peace and acceptance for their Self also. It's a gift to our Self and others, a very powerful gift. No more, no less is required here.

We look to our relationships to find our happiness and once again, if we're coming from a place where happiness is within us, our relationships are often positive and smooth. When we're not coming from that core happiness within us, our relationships are often disappointing and frustrating.

We look to our relationships to balance out what we don't have within ourselves, and this is quite an unrealistic expectation in most cases. This would explain why many relationships don't last. They will always fall short of the expectation if we have that shortfall within ourselves.

The most important relationship we can have is the relationship with our Self. When that relationship with our Self is strong and grounded, when we look to external sources for relationships, such as friendships, life partners, intimacy, then we're not looking for external validation. What we're looking for is someone to share our journey with. When we release the expectation within the relationship and accept that person 100% as they are, then the relationship has an opportunity to flourish, blossom and grow rather than to wither and die.

If we look back over our relationships throughout our lifetime, and see what sort of reflection and message we are receiving from these relationships, we may see the areas that we want to heal and consolidate within ourselves. That which we see as lacking in the other person, is often what we're lacking within ourselves, and that person and that relationship is often reflecting that. So once again, within ourselves, when we learn to love ourselves unconditionally, we'll find that happiness externally as well.

Life is meant to be shared and yes we do come into our life and this world on our own, and leave on our own, but it's the relationships in our life that can add that extra colour, the nuances, the different shades. It's an opportunity to see life from another perspective outside of our own.

Rather than trying to make these relationships a reflection of ourselves, or a shadow of ourselves, what if we could see these relationships as new ways of looking at the world, as new opportunities for growth and to add another dimension, or colour, to the world through somebody else's eyes? It's quite special to be able to do that. It's like being in the presence of a child, and you see the child's joy and excitement at every new experience. When we're in the presence of that child, we feel that joy, that freshness of seeing the world through those new eyes, and being part of that is a gift.

Each relationship we have, we have that opportunity; to see the world through someone else's eyes, and at the same time retain our own identity. Often in relationships we release our identity and amalgamate with the other person, and this loss of Self takes us away from that core happiness. So if we can retain that sense of Self whilst also appreciating and enjoying the perspective of the other person, then we end up with a full, enriched, abundant life.

Relationships can serve many purposes. We have relationships with parental figures, with our children, siblings, work colleagues, relatives, lovers, partners, friends. Our whole world, being filled with people, of course, is all about relationships. So within the dynamics of all these varying shades of communication and perspectives, to be able to retain our sense of Self is vital, if we are to move fluidly and smoothly within these different relationships.

It can be very comforting for other people to be in the presence of someone who has a strong sense of Self. It feels very solid and warm, and encompasses the people and things around. Everybody has that sense of Self, it's just about remembering that we need to go within to find that sense of Self, that our external relationships are not going to give us that. The most important relationship is with our Self.

Meditation: Relationships

To connect with our relationship with our Self, we're going to focus on our inner being, our heart centre. So once again, concentrating and bringing your attention to your breathing, the breath as it rises and it falls. Bringing this breath into your heart centre, expand that heart centre, and energising it, until it radiates out to everything, and everyone around.

There may be a relationship that you have that is particularly dear to you, or there may be a relationship that needs healing. Once again, create that heart image in your heart centre. Fill it with a colour that you choose, or that you feel is needed for this relationship. Gently place a picture of that person or people into that heart image, encompassing it with the warmth and beauty of the colour that you have chosen.

Once that heart is encompassing that relationship, extend a rainbow from the heart in your heart centre up to your head, taking a copy of that heart image with that relationship within it, up to your head and clicking it into place. Click!

Connect your heart and your mind to encompass all thoughts, feelings and emotions in this beautiful colour and this beautiful shape. Knowing that this is safely in place, and you can recall that picture at any time and bring warmth, healing and happiness to you, gently open your eyes and come back into the room when you're ready.

My Human Experience: Our Children and Family

Again, the topic of our children could be a whole book in itself but for the purposes here, I'll keep it short, but maybe not so sweet.

This is one area of my life that has involved my most extreme growth. Giving birth to my son Daniel, was my first experience of unconditional love. It was both exquisite and painful as I held him in my arms. My battered emotional state was not well equipped to cope with the strength of the love I had for him and still do. My successful career as Head of Department of Music at a Secondary School, went completely out the window without a second thought, and nothing mattered more than him. My twelve month maternity leave was extended permanently. Also for my beautiful daughter Jessica, who was born twenty months later. They were my best friends, my soul mates, my shining lights in a somewhat grim family life.

I am sad to say, that after years of being in a volatile marriage and going through a very hostile divorce, those two beautiful souls are changed beyond recognition. If I had known then what I know now, I would have taken them out of that environment sooner, and protected them from all that life should not expose them to. The journey of forgiveness towards myself has been immense, painful and multi-layered. Finally, the understanding that they are on their own journey has given me some peace of mind.

Allowing them to move through whatever it is they need to, has been one of my biggest challenges in life, while retaining my personal boundaries within that. Like many parents, if I could re-write events and choices, my life and theirs may have been very different, but that not being possible, I can only forgive myself and others. In doing so, I have found some measure of peace.

What gives me hope for my relationship with my children, is when I reflect back on myself as that hurt child and adult, and how I blamed everything and everyone for my unhappiness. Now I have this amazing relationship with my Mum, and blame has gone from my mind. It wasn't always the case, and a few years ago Mum, who is very spiritually aware, said with absolute dread that we had better sort our relationship out as otherwise we would have to come back and face each other in another lifetime. Luckily for both of us I think our work here is done, and we enjoy good times and good conversations together, which I would never have predicted years ago.

As my children are now experiencing being parents themselves, I hope they discover unconditional love and forgiveness also and find it in their hearts to realise life is not predictable and guaranteed. How we handle the difficult times is more important than expecting life to be a smooth road ahead. In gaining that resilience they may move to a place of understanding.

In my work with clients and workshop participants, I have discovered that when you scratch the surface, most families have some level of dysfunction, and hiding it in shame only perpetuates it. I used to be so ashamed of my perceived failures as a mother but now realise it has enabled me to truly understand the plight of others and be able to help them. When I was going through some of my toughest hours with my kids, ironically I was also doing voluntary work running a parent's Toughlove support group at night and through the day working with 'at risk' teens who had been kicked out of the school system and sometimes home. Working with both parents and children and getting both perspectives helped me realise that everyone has their own reality of life and events, all valid in their own right.

Message: Our Children and Family

These relationships we have with our children and family are sometimes the most fraught or volatile. The interplay of different characteristics and personalities can create opportunities for growth, but also can, in certain circumstances, be very distressful.

These relationships that we've chosen in this lifetime, that play out as dramas and interchange and interplay of characters and scenarios, can lead to intoxicating love, pure unconditional love at its best, and at its worst deep distress, disharmony and disease. This dis-ease that sometimes occurs with our children or even any other member of our family, can take on a life force of its own and become all consuming and overpowering.

If we remember that a parent is a vessel for bringing children into this world, then we can understand that we each have our own responsibility to, and relationship with, our true Self. Amongst the interchange and interplay of personalities, we must retain this.

Although these child/parent relationships are opportunities for growth, and are vital in our lives, we must at the same time retain our own identity, independently of that relationship with our child or parent. Otherwise, our identity is threatened to become a reflection or a manifestation of that relationship. Our identity becomes contingent on what sort of relationship we have with our children or parents. Ideally when all our lessons are learned from each other, we can enjoy beautiful pure unconditional relationships, and that's our goal. But on that journey, in attaining that, if we lose our sense of our identity, it is unlikely that we will achieve that unconditional relationship.

So once again it comes back to our relationship with our Self. First and foremost, to make sure that it is intact, strong and grounded. In having this, it becomes a platform for our relationship with our children or parents. Whether that relationship is going through a time of dis-array or dis-ease, we still have that strong base. This base is not just for us, but it also creates that platform and solidity for our children, or other family members, to know that we are there for them when and if they need us.

As parents, our children have their own lives and their own lessons to learn, and our responsibility as a parent is to hold that space for them to be able to learn and experience whatever it is they need to experience in this lifetime. If we interfere and try and help them with their lessons to such an extent that they no longer are able to learn their own strengths, then in fact we are doing them a disservice. In holding that space for them we are there for them if we are needed, but not to take over and learn their lessons for them. As a parent this can be the hardest part of this relationship, holding that space and seeing how it plays out for them.

Meditation: Our Children and Family

Closing your eyes and bringing your attention to the breath as it rises and it falls, paying particular attention to that breath energising your heart centre. Expand that heart centre, creating that beautiful heart image in the centre, choosing any colour that you need, to heal this relationship. With that beautiful colour embedded in your heart centre, bring a picture of your loved one or loved ones into that heart centre, bathed in that colour and that light. Breathe deeply into that heart centre, bathing those people and those loved ones in this colour, and this feeling of unconditional love. Now, creating a copy of that picture and that heart, take it up through a rainbow of light and colour, up into your head and click it into place. Click!

This connection between heart and head with regards to this relationship, is bringing it balance, harmony and ultimately joy, to allow this relationship to manifest in whatever way is right for this relationship. Whatever that relationship holds, we have this connection and are always connected to this and to our connection to Self.

With this connection firmly in place, coming from that place of unconditional love for our Self and others, gently open your eyes when you're ready, and come back into the room.

Chapter 3
Health & Wellbeing

"Everything I need to know is revealed to me. Everything I need comes to me"

–Louise Hay: Heal Your Body

My Human Experience

The most important thing I have learned recently is to listen to my body and how it is responding in certain situations whether it be around certain foods, people or environments. It sounds so simple yet I wonder if many illnesses come from people being disconnected to what their body is telling them. An animal or young child knows exactly what is going on with them and will move towards or away from whatever it is.

We, as adults, often override our intuition and then wonder why we become unhappy and ill. I have come to realise that the body is an amazing tool, instead of seeing it as a burden. Many people on their spiritual path see their body as an encumbrance when we can instead see it as a wonderful vehicle of awareness for our journey in this lifetime. Not to mention all the fun we can have with it of course.

When my father left, I was about age 10 and I manifested rheumatic fever which is a heart condition. Louise Hay with Heal Your Life, later became my companion in working out the source emotion and thought pattern and, as always, her connection of our physical ailments to our emotional source, is so enlightening. I had a heart murmur for years and recently when I went to the doctors for a check up, found it had gone. I put that down to the heart centred healing I have been doing recently. How cool is that to be able to heal our own body?

Later in my life, when there was a lot of trauma around the birth of my first grandchild, I manifested ovarian cysts as a direct response to the emotions I was experiencing. Luckily I had amazing people around me, one of which worked with me around my beliefs and emotional pain. The cysts expelled before needing surgery, in fact no more than 30 minutes after one of the sessions. We hadn't even been working around the issue of the cysts, but when the clutter of the emotions and mind cleared away, so did the imbalance in my body. I am truly in awe of what we are capable of achieving.

Being able to express my emotions rather than suppress them has helped keep me in good health throughout my life. Sometimes it's very messy, but my body is grateful I'm sure. Even better would be to stay calm and peaceful in the face of all life's daily challenges. I'm still working on that one, but it is definitely getting easier. Ironically the calmer I remain, the less challenges present themselves. That good old friend, the paradox of change, always makes me laugh at myself and my human manoeuvrings.

Trying to explain the paradox of change to people is challenging as it is appears to be a backwards concept. In order to have what you want you have to be comfortable without having it. Figure that out. I guess it's all about what you're directing your attention to, and if it is to that which you don't want, then you just keep on getting more of what you don't want. Or vice versa, so it does actually make sense from an energy perspective to determine where you're putting your focus. I love that it also removes fear and attachment to 'things' and people as that can lead to unhealthy dependence which benefits no-one in the end.

When I was younger I had friends who were sick a lot and I wondered why I didn't get sick. That was before I understood the mind/body connection and I thought it was like a handout of cards and my quota was being saved up for the big one, like the big C, cancer. Back then I was unaware of how we subconsciously create illness ourselves. Sometimes, I noticed with my friends, that it was the only time they really allowed themselves to take time off and rest, apart from sleeping at night of course. Sometimes it was the only time they received love and attention, so you can see the positive payoff we sometimes receive from being unwell.

The concept of the illness being a messenger is one that I find very intriguing and again, it really challenges the mind to come to terms with that; honestly take the message that is presenting via the illness, make the changes, and subsequently heal. Sometimes bad things do just seem to happen as in the case of children and good people dying unexpectedly and, from a spiritual perspective, I have come to see death as not something to fear but something that is part of a bigger picture. If we regard death as final, then that is pretty scary but if we consider that maybe this lifetime is just one of many, then death takes on a whole new meaning. Other cultures seem to have a much better grasp on death than our western cultures, which are largely fear based. Some cultures celebrate the life and passing over, and I think that is a really great way to also live your life, in celebration of each day.

With my brother and father now passed over, I did wonder at the time, if I was denying and avoiding grief but I seemed to have a sense that this wasn't the end. I have had several visits from them in my dreams and often sense them around me, keeping an eye on things.

The inward turning of emotions is a chemical cocktail, as many people now understand. The medical profession used to describe it as nonsense that stress created illnesses and it is now accepted knowledge, thankfully. I saw my brother whom I loved very much, fester with frustration and unexpressed anger and die from cancer. Because my Dad had been an overtly angry man, at some time my brother, sensitive soul that he was, decided he would never do that and suppressed any 'undesirable' emotions such as anger. To be able to express what we are feeling in a non damaging way is such a gift to ourselves and others in the maintaining of a healthy equilibrium. The simple daily ritual of thinking of things I'm grateful for at the end of each day, and on waking, things I'm looking forward to, is enough to direct me towards a new direction. It's so easy otherwise to fall into victimhood.

Like many women, the women in my family have food and eating issues and I have had a number of clients also with this. Knowing that our bodies are expressions of all aspects of us, when in protection or in need of comfort emotionally, we pad up and I've come to realise that when all is well with emotional and spiritual issues, the body is automatically in alignment. Weight becomes a non issue. Isn't that so wonderful to know that we are in charge of our health and able to keep clearing away the debris of life.

I've always been pretty comfortable with my body but recently tried to drop a few kilos, however I put on many more. With the work I do I knew I must have hit a nerve in the subconscious so that has been very insightful. I realised that after all these years I was still in protection from childhood and relationship stuff. I also figure that when a challenge comes up in my own life, it is an opportunity and a gift to understand it more, and then to be able to help my clients with similar challenges. Recognizing that everything in life is a mirror, I've noticed that when I'm working through something, I attract clients and people into my life with similar challenges.

It is all a work in progress and when I look back at all the different therapies and modalities I have learned, used and received, they are all absolutely what I needed at the time. There is no one solution for everyone and with such an abundance of amazing modalities and processes out there to assist us on our journey of wellbeing, we are spoilt for choice. I believe there is no better time to be alive and participating in this. The synchronicities are abundant as people, books, classes, or whatever you need comes into your life at exactly the right time. All we have to do is stay open and allow them in.

The array of modalities to learn out there is such a feast. After learning each one that I have been drawn to, I have experienced a significant shift each time, confirming it was the right step to take. I went through a phase in my forties where I started getting into some pretty 'out there' spiritual experiences and had an episode one night where I tapped into something malevolent, or so I thought at the time. I couldn't wake up out of my nightmare and lost about two years of memory, my mind just shutting down. Since then I am a bit more careful about the types of people and tools I bring into my field.

It is only recently, ten years later, that I am now allowing spiritual practices to re-enter my life. As I am now more grounded and in alignment with my mind, body, spirit, I have had some beautiful experiences with this. The most recent of these has been the receiving of the messages and meditations from my Higher Self to help heal my own life and to share with others. I feel truly blessed in my life to have experienced this, as can anyone when they are ready. I think that is the key, as I know people who have tried and tried to do things with no luck and when they're relaxed, and in a state of open allowing, then whatever needs to happen will.

From my observations of my own life, my family, friends, and clients, I have noticed that so many of the current problems they are having are coming from that hurt child. Regardless of their age or current position in life, it mostly seems to go back to those early years and, of course, we now know through research why that is. Knowing this and changing it are two quite different issues. Releasing those childhood wounds and hurts is vital to help us grow as a person in every way. I am so excited now to be able to share such an easy way of releasing those old hurts. The change processes I was using prior to the heart centred healing were quite complex and even teaching them, could create more complexity in people's lives instead of simplifying their lives. I am hopeful that with easier ways of accessing our own innate power to heal, more people will be the change they seek in the world, thank you Gandhi!

Message: Clearing Unwanted Thoughts & Feelings

Of the thoughts we have, which are the thoughts that belong to us, that are from us, and which thoughts are simply part of the overlays and accumulations of experiences, and other peoples' opinions and expressions? Which thoughts are intrinsic to us?

There are so many thoughts running around in our head at any given time, how do we know which thoughts to take notice of and which thoughts to ignore? So as these thoughts pass through our mind, as we notice them, what do we notice about them? How do these thoughts make us feel? Do these thoughts make us feel good about ourselves and other people and other things or do they make us feel bad about ourselves, other people and other things? Quite simply in noticing how these thoughts make us feel, we can identify and know them as ours or something other than us. In simply noticing this, this is enough to dispel any doubt about the quality of these thoughts.

People often identify with these thoughts as being themselves and most often these thoughts have nothing to do with us but everything to do with everyone else and everything else. In which case, we need to question whether we really want to identify with these thoughts, when they are not actually about us and for us and of us.

So what to do with these thoughts? We notice them. We identify them as being either our thoughts or somebody else's that we have taken on at some point in our life. What do we do with these thoughts now, once we have done this? Do we want to have other people's thoughts within us? Is this helpful to us?

It is up to us to decide whether we want to have those thoughts within us or send them away with love. We choose what thoughts we have within us. We have to decide if we want to have that thought pattern running through us continuously as part of our Being, or whether we choose to dissolve that thought, no longer to be run through our Being.

In doing so we get to choose the quality of our life, as many people's lives are identified and expressed from a thought about themselves, or another person or something around them, even about their world. We can identify and choose this quality of life that we are now going to have around us and within us. This is the most powerful choice that we can make about our lives. We are in charge of making those choices at any point in time thus creating our own world, our own life, our own Being.

So how to identify and make these choices and bring about this reality whatever it is we are choosing? The following meditation is for clearing unwanted thoughts and feelings.

Meditation: Clearing Unwanted Thoughts & Feelings

Closing your eyes and bringing your attention to the breath as it rises and it falls, expanding that heart centre in the centre of our chest area, filling that area with energy. As we breathe with our attention in our heart centre, we take a thought as it comes through our mind. We take that thought from our mind and bring it down through a rainbow of light for cleansing and purifying. Regardless of what that thought is, whether it currently gives us pleasure or gives us pain, we bring that thought down into the heart centre and we bathe it in a colour, whatever colour comes through to encircle and encompass that thought.

As it's bathed in that beautiful colour in our heart centre, we can even create a heart around that thought. Being in our heart centre, the centre of our Being, we intrinsically know the quality and the relevance of this thought, whether it be of us or of someone else, or something else. In bathing this thought with that beautiful colour, that thought is automatically integrated as part of our Being in a healthy, heart-felt way that will enhance our Being. Whatever has had to be transformed about that thought has been transformed, bringing us love and happiness regardless of where it came from. That thought that we originally had is no longer as it was. It has now been transformed into whatever it needs to be for our highest goal. It cannot bring us anything except love and happiness now.

Each time we have a thought and we're curious about whether that thought is from us or from somewhere else, or something else, we simply need to bring our breathing into our heart centre. Then bring that thought down through a beautiful rainbow of colour into your heart centre for integration or transformation so that there is no such thing anymore as a bad thought. It is simply a thought that is waiting to be transformed and released or transformed and integrated, whichever is in our best interests.

We can trust that our Inner Soul, our Inner Being has that wisdom and will make that decision. Nothing will be lost that is necessary for us at this point in time. Anything that we need at any point in time can be transformed into a state where we can take it and receive the goodness and happiness from it.

Knowing that we can now do this at any time with any thought, just come back into the room when you're ready and gently opening your eyes.

My Human Experience: Releasing Addictions & Energies

This chapter was added as an afterthought, as at first I thought this was an area that I had no direct experience of myself, apart from witnessing the powerful grip that drugs had on my son. When I looked at the underlying reasons for addictions, particularly when working with clients with addictions, I realised the addiction of choice may vary as do the underlying reasons. Respecting my client's privacy, I choose not to comment too much on this but really I was not so different from them.

My addiction of choice was busyness. I actually had to look in the dictionary to see if this was in fact a word, how it was spelt and what it meant. One of the descriptions was 'cluttered with detail to the point of being distracting'. That sounds really silly and strange, but on consideration, it was just another way of avoiding being still and quiet with myself.

We know that addictions can be to anything; food, alcohol, drugs, sex, relationships, pornography, gambling, sports, a person, relationships etc, etc, the list goes on and on. Each addiction is simply a way of distracting ourselves from some underlying hurt or pain. It takes away the pain of our reality, a hurt sometimes so deep that we are often unaware of what it is and where it came from. The addiction can mask and cover over feelings of loneliness, inadequacy, fear, sadness and, once again, the list can go on and on.

The emotions that we have in response to experiences and situations are sometimes too hard for people to bear. I have also seen people use addictions as a way of bringing excitement into an otherwise dull life as they don't have the confidence to move into their own power and joy.

There is no point in taking away the substance or object of the addiction unless these underlying reasons for the addiction are met. Otherwise the person will only pick up another addiction, which could even be worse. I have seen this happen with the people around me. It is like a blind person stumbling towards or away from something but they don't know what.

I always professed I was high on life. A great idea and probably at times I was, but when I really got honest with myself which, of course, is always the first challenge, I realised my manic busyness was a way of avoiding deep underlying hurt. Not wanting to dig up old stuff, I have used other processes to resolve this and the meditations I was given were such a blessing, when of course I take the time to do them. Changing some of my limiting beliefs about myself and others has also helped me move to a place of calm, peace and acceptance. Now, when I notice myself start to get 'busy' I stop and check what is going on and take the steps to release whatever it is that is pushing that need.

To think I would be let of so lightly would seem a bit arrogant and sure enough, I recently visited a medical intuitive, and discovered that my system was in chaos at a very deep core level from trying to keep control over my emotions. Sometimes you don't know what you don't know and in this case, what I had thought of as clearing my emotions, had in fact been kindergarten for my system. I had built up such a strong protective layer that my body and energy field was seriously under stress, trying to 'hold it all together' and avoid the pain. My blood pressure was 'boiling up' in response to my suppressed emotions and Louise Hay's A to Z directory, 'Heal Your Body' confirms this. The symptom of high blood pressure was giving me a clear message that all was not well. As described earlier, I had become very adept at repressing my emotions which is a deadly cocktail. I guess you could say I had become an emotional control freak. Control was my way of avoiding the painful emotions without using external substances but creating a lot of damage internally to my system nonetheless.

As mentioned in the previous chapter, I have recently experienced some dramatic changes in my personal relationship. Once again the paradox of the universe was at play. While I was busy receiving spiritual downloads, my partner was busy downloading things of quite a different nature, if you get my meaning. Through some seemingly random synchronicities, I discovered my partner of six years had quite a serious addiction.

All my experience working with clients with addictions did nothing to reduce the incredible betrayal and hurt I felt. It has taken some time to realise it was in fact a blessing in disguise as it served to bring up old feelings of abandonment and not feeling good enough that I needed to address. I went through the myriad of emotions and I did notice that I moved quickly through them to arrive at a place of acceptance and compassion. In the past that would have taken me years, not weeks or months to arrive at.

What this highlighted, more-so than the event, was the lack of open and honest communication, connection and respect in the relationship, which had been the original reason I had stopped living with him several years earlier.

If my sense of Self had been stronger, I know I wouldn't have had to go through this final event and suffer as I did, as there had been many signs along the way that I chose to ignore. I was short cutting both of us by not allowing him to sort his own life out. It was a hard lesson learnt but one that I won't forget in a hurry.

Forgive but don't forget!

We are each on our own journey and it serves neither of us well if I keep going in, thinking I can help 'fix' things up. It only shortcuts both of our growth.

The messages and meditations have been a God send to help me through those dark nights of the soul.

What a journey it has been and one which continues to present opportunities for insight and growth.

I am now able to offer support as a friend without losing myself in his problems.

Message: Releasing Addictions & Energies

When there is a dis-connect with other energies, it can create a fragmented state. This disconnect from other energies could be when we're connecting with someone with a different energy frequency or it can occur when we choose to disconnect from someone. It can create a fracture in one or both energy fields. Whatever the reason for this disconnect, the important point here is that there may need to be some healing to smooth over this fractured area in the energy field. If left disconnected this can result in difficult mental states and even dis-ease within the body as a result of this disconnect.

How do we know when there's a dis-connect? What does this experience feel like? Being in a physical form in this lifetime we can experience it as a physical discomfort. It could sit as a feeling of discomfort in the area around the solar plexus, the seat of the emotion or in any other part of the body that is relevant to the relationship that is being affected by the disconnect.

This disconnect can also be experienced as an extreme emotional response as we experience anything from despair to rage depending on which end of the disconnect you're on. To avoid it being cataclysmic in response to this disconnect, it is important to heal it at the deepest level and smooth back the energy field to a place of harmony and peace that we all seek.

We can experience disconnection in some or all areas of our lives. It can be a disconnect from our emotions, a disconnect from a person, or people, or group. It can be a disconnect to an energy force, even to our soul. When we experience this disconnect in our daily lives, our lives are punctuated by disharmony, dis-ease and chaotic events occurring in our life. Although on one level we don't want this chaos and this disconnect, on another level, it is protecting us from that which we don't know, or that which we have forgotten, which is our connection to Self.

To reconnect to that deeper level of being, we connect to our inner Self, which is connected to the source. We cannot have a connection and disconnection at the same time, so when we choose to go through this process to reconnect and heal our disconnection, then health and harmony are restored into our life, and ultimately happiness within.

What is happiness? Happiness is an absence of disconnection, of dis-ease, of dis-harmony, to be replaced with joy and calm and peace within. Disconnection can be on one or many levels but it is all one and the same. When we are not connected we don't have access to all those wondrous things we seek.

The paradox is that when disconnected we seek happiness through many other means, through addictive behaviours and artificial substances. We are in fact seeking that same place of joy that we have when we are connected, but in seeking this connection, in this way, we are in fact pushing ourselves further away from connection, purely to experience it fleetingly. We don't realise that we can have access to this connection all the time as our normal state of being.

Once the realisation is there, how do we reconnect with our inner joy, calm and peace? How do we disconnect from our own and other's conflict, and from external and internal interferences?'

Meditation: Releasing Addictions & Energies

Close your eyes, and focus on your breathing. Notice your breath as it rises and it falls. Allow that breath, that life force energy to flow through you freely. As you breathe, bring your breath and attention into your heart centre, activating that life force energy. As you allow that heart centre to fill with the life force, choose a colour to support this process, any colour that you choose, or are given or receive.

Allowing this colour, this colour of connection, to spread slowly throughout your body, filling your abdomen, your arms, and your hands all the way down through your torso and your legs, down to your feet and at the same time extending up through your throat, and filling your head, your ears, your mouth, your nose until every part of your being is filled with this luxuriant colour.

As you feel this throughout your body, allow it to move and pulsate with every cell in your body, creating a shimmering that extends from your body out into your field to help heal and connect all those people around you who come into contact with you, and feel this connection to Self and Source as they move freely in and out of your presence. This energy and colour, flowing and pulsating through your body, is there at any time and all times, to access your connection to Self.

Know that all external substances and energies that have previously been required to experience this sensation are no longer necessary. You have all that is required within you to access pure joy, happiness and peace. When you're ready, bring that focus, and all that shimmering energy, and concentrate that into the heart centre to be stored and accessed at any time, at all times resonating within you and out of you. As both an internal resource and an external resource and protection from any external influences that you no longer choose to have in your life.

Knowing that this is now yours and you have access to this at all times, bring your breathing gently back down into the heart centre. When you're ready, gently open your eyes and come back into the room.

Message: Healing Our Body

Why is it that our body is often seen as an encumbrance, a burden, an imperfection?

Why are we often discontent about our body, disconnected, dis-satisfied, dis-eased?

Our body is the vessel in this lifetime. It is our chosen vehicle of expression. We choose at a level beyond consciousness to have this body to bring us whatever lessons we decide to learn in this lifetime. Within repeated family patterns, these can be lessons learned directly or indirectly through our family and their relationships to their bodies also.

How we feel about our bodies is an expression of how we feel about ourselves at a much deeper level. While we stay focussed on our bodies we are limited to the body. The body will never be perfect due to the very nature of the material it is made of and its declining process. Yet at the same time it is a perfect mechanism for us to achieve awareness of what is happening at a much deeper level. If the body is a messenger, are we listening to the message it is giving us at any given time? Even the simple message of 'Have we had enough food', 'Are we comfortable with that person?', 'Is there something in my body that needs to rest?' Our body is the most accurate messenger for us of what is happening to us right now. But are we listening?

To go beyond the body and its limitations, we must first master the craft of being fully aware of our body. Once this craft is perfected, it becomes part of our innate being to be aware and we can then transcend the constant attention that we normally have to pay to our body. If we observe animals in nature, they are perfectly tuned in to their body and its requirements and its messages. They eat when hungry, stop when full, sleep when tired, play when playful, run when scared. As humans, we have suppressed these basic instincts and it is at the expense of our body's health and wellbeing.

How to remedy this and restore our body to its natural state of health and wellbeing?

Meditation: Healing Our Body

Close your eyes and bring your attention to the breath. Notice as it rises and falls. Bring this breath into the heart centre, allowing it to expand and energise the heart centre. As you bring your breath and attention to the heart centre, allow a colour to fill the heart centre. This colour is the carrier of this message that we are about to receive. Allow the colour in your heart centre to expand and spread out around your body, slowly and steadily and as it moves slowly throughout your body, notice any areas where the colour changes. It may deepen or lighten, or even miss areas in your body as it slowly fills your arms, hands, throat, head, ears, trunk, lower body, legs and feet.

Allow this colour to settle and gently rock in your body setting up a ripple effect. As this colour ripples throughout your body, allow it to move into those areas that were previously empty or lighter. Stay with these areas until they are flowing freely. Allow the colours that were deeper or darker in certain areas to ripple and clear, dispersing any blockages or density within your body. Continue this process moving through every area of your body until your body ripples and shimmers in one continuous and even colour.

Allow this colour to brighten with good health and well being, shimmering and sending out that shimmer to your outer body, encompassing many levels of being. This is your natural, healthy state of being. Know that this can continue and will continue and you can restore this at anytime. Gently bring your attention and breathing back to your heart centre and come back into the room, opening your eyes when you're ready.

Chapter 4

Career or Calling

"Have the courage to follow your heart and intuition. They somehow already know what you truly want to become. Everything else is secondary."

–Steve Jobs

My Human Experience

This is an area of my life where I have a lot of experience, if you call having lots of careers and jobs, experience. This includes; working in KFC, weeding traffic islands, teaching music and piano, driving trucks, selling insurance, being Head of Department of Music in a Secondary School, setting up and running a farm recruitment agency, teaching children with learning difficulties, packing shelves in the supermarket, helping 'at risk' teenagers into work, Career Consultant in a Tertiary Institute, Wellness Coach in private practice, International Instructor! Whew! There are many more, too many to count, but as you can see there doesn't seem to be a system to it at all.

Every one of these jobs and careers, I have been extremely grateful for as it was just what I needed at the time. This seemingly random collection has in fact made complete sense at each stage in my life and was what I needed to experience, as I came to realise in retrospect.

I used to think that these opportunities that come our way in life at different times were just chance but now with the work I do, I have come to realise that there is no such thing as chance and the synchronicities or meaningful coincidences are in fact part of our pathway. Of course we always have the freewill to take them up and in many cases for people that is free won't. When I look back I can actually see that it was in fact a fine tuned pathway to where I am right now.

One job I haven't mentioned in that list was my stint at working for the Inland Revenue, aged 17, straight out of school. Good old Mum found that job for me and I absolutely loathed it. I pity the people who had their returns in at the time I was there, as I had no idea what I was doing, being one of these creative types—great excuse. I have great respect for the people who work there though, as it is quite challenging working with numbers all day. Well, for me anyway. But I'm sure it lights some people up depending on their personality type. It served its purpose though, because as soon as I'd saved enough money I jumped the ditch to Australia. I don't think I even told Mum, who later confided she never thought she'd see me again. I'm sure there were moments when that was quite a comforting thought as I'd been a very troublesome teenager with all that anger and hurt bottled up, waiting for a loving, supporting person such as her to dump it on.

Anyway, after a year of doing odd jobs and enjoying the Sydney lifestyle, I was dragged back by Mum and my piano teacher to go to university to study music. I really didn't enjoy that at all, not realising at the time that I was following Mum's dream, not mine. The silver lining was the arts papers I was allowed to study, including archaeology and psychology, both of which I was fascinated by. Years later they came to the fore again so not all wasted time there.

I come from a long line of teachers, my mother, my grandmother. I'm not sure past there, but it feels like a long line especially when as a teenager I resisted everything about my family. When I finally realised that I loved teaching, my music and piano playing led me down the path of teaching little children how to play music. I found that I really loved to share knowledge, and loved being around kids for their simplicity, and their naturalness. I spent many years teaching in many different ways, working with teens, which everyone thought I was crazy to do but again I loved their humour, their quirkiness, and music being a creative subject was an easy one to share as everyone has a natural rhythm in them.

These careers that we seem to slip into, or maybe it is that they've been programmed into us, can sometimes be exactly what we need. Sometimes we resist that and go to the extreme opposite polarity to resist that programming. As a career consultant I really tried to emphasise that when you're truly authentic with what you're doing for your living then you never have to work a day in your life. There are so many people dragging through life staying in a career or job for security. I've found that when I'm doing what lights me up it also brings joy to others so everyone benefits. Being a 'leap of faith' kind of gal, I have had no problem leaving when this stops and each time, after the initial abyss of the unknown, it has always had a better outcome than if I had stayed for security.

Helping people make career decisions in my role as a career consultant, I came to realise that the biggest impediment to them getting to where they wanted to get to was actually their own self imposed barriers. This is what led me to the study of the mind and how to remove some of those limiting beliefs and barriers. This fascinating work is still part of my private coaching practice as well as the new material that has been coming through. In making career choices it's important to note that the best choice right now might be quite different than in five or ten years time. What feels right now is what is important. Long term career planning is important also, but if getting there means years of pain and struggle, I would question this as there are plenty of careers where the pathway is enjoyable and flowing, when it's the right choice for you. As we each have our own perspective on situations and events, it is up to us to find the pathway that best suits us and not others.

Working with clients now in my coaching work, I have noticed that many people retain the residual damage from schooling, resulting in low self esteem and social anxiety issues. This is more prevalent than people realise and having been a teacher I feel the shame of this profession. As an example, teachers in the past were ill equipped to deal with dyslexia and these amazing picture thinkers have had to struggle through school, not realising it was not their disability but a teaching disability that prevented them learning as easily as they could. The labels of ADD (attention deficit disorder) and ADHD (attention deficit hyperactivity disorder) are often bestowed on students who are kinaesthetic learners and ill suited to the restricted confines of a predominantly left brained education system. Labels, while useful for explaining clusters of behaviour, can have a hugely detrimental effect on the individual as happened with my son at age eight, when he was told by the school that he was ADHD. He went from being a happy, high functioning boy, to an angry, defiant student after only a couple of years in the education system. Despite my best efforts at trying to reassure him, not to measure himself as a person by a spelling or maths test, he remained unconvinced. Extra help and learning only seemed to reinforce his belief that he wasn't good enough and his resulting angry behaviour attracted a lot of adverse attention and still does. I hope that he will one day remember how amazing he really is and heal the hurts from this part of his life.

Many of the criminal behavioural issues we are seeing in our society come from learning difficulties at school that haven't been addressed properly. The impact on people's lives is immense and though teachers are doing the best they can with the resources they have, it is unfortunate that so many people are impacted. It seems these people can go one of two ways, either ending up in the prison system or CEO of their own company. Sometimes there is a fine line between the two. Many of the greatest entrepreneurs that I have met, struggled at school but have far surpassed their classmates due to having their thinking 'out of the box'. This seems to work in their favour later in life but they often still carry the stigma of their alternative learning style. They have had to become more resourceful to achieve things rather than following the mainstream way. Again, it is being able to move beyond the hurt child to remember who they truly are and find what lights them up. Hats off to them!

Career choices are often made from a limited knowledge of what is out there and I would strongly encourage people to do the research and look around at all the different career options there are, that are hidden away behind the public eye. There are some fascinating careers out there that receive little recognition. What I have found is that one of the most important keys in choosing a successful career is recognizing what environment you like to work in, whether that be with nature, finance, health, retail, animals, sports etc. Which environment makes you feel energised and excited rather than depleted?

Sometimes it's the people you are working with that make it all worthwhile. One of the fun jobs I remember was being all together in a room with other university students, opening envelopes for share certificates. An incredibly boring activity doing this, but the conversations that we had were incredible. It was an environment of high energy and lively minds. Mind you, it was only for a month which was probably as long as the stories and conversation would have lasted. Some of the best jobs in terms of what I was actually doing became heavily laden with despair due to being around toxic environments and people.

I became quite fascinated by how and why people move around in their careers and did my post graduate qualifications in Career Development; whether there is a system to it or if it is random selection, a bit like choosing a mate? Pondering on whether there was in fact any method in it all, I can see that what is a seemingly random and unrelated career step at the time can hold you in good stead later. Volunteer work is an example of this and I would highly recommend this for someone getting back into work or even starting out in the work force, to help gain confidence and build new skills. It is low pressure and you usually get a lot out of it, though not in monetary terms at first.

At one stage I did quite a lot of volunteer work in areas I felt passionately about or felt there was a need. One of these was facilitating a Toughlove parent's support group as there had been an absence of support in the countryside where I lived. At the time I was going to hell and back with my troublesome teens. Seeing other parents arriving on the brink of despair and breakdown and seeing them a few weeks later when they had regained their personal power back was incredibly gratifying.

It was quite funny though as when they arrived they all seemed to think they were going to find ways to sort out these blights in their household, only to find out that it was in fact themselves that had to change. I can still see the look of shock on their faces but then the incredulous looks when they came back the next week to report the changes in their household. Be the change you seek in the world as Gandhi so aptly put it.

While I was studying by correspondence, I had another volunteer job working with 'at risk' teens who had been kicked out of the school system. These kids had some pretty serious chips on their shoulders but were in fact lots of fun as soon as they realised I was there to help them, not lecture them. Getting them into work where they could build their self esteem back up was the key, and it was so gratifying to see them turn their lives around.

So all this voluntary work duly noted on my CV was actually what clinched me securing my dream job as a Career Consultant after having been out of the workforce for years while parenting. Of course I had done all the relevant study as well but volunteer work was a great transition step into paid employment. For people wanting to move into their dream career or chosen calling, I would highly recommend finding some related voluntary work as a first step, as it is beneficial to all concerned. It is also a fantastic way to feel worthwhile and valued in our sometimes lonely western society.

Another area in careers that I feel very strongly about is when to leave your job or career. Being a 'leap of faith' type of person as mentioned before, I have tended to take this option. It has always worked for me but isn't for everyone. In one job, actually my dream job, I realised it was time to leave when I was driving to work and found myself hoping I would have a car crash rather than face what I saw at the time was a highly stressful workplace bullying situation. Having come from years of living with abuse, I had a very low threshold for what I perceived as bullying. I realise now, they were just dealing with their own insecurities, as I have never been a conformer and that is quite scary for some people. Rather than work it through I would always do a rapid stage exit left, as if I was fleeing for my life. I guess that is why many of my most successful career steps have been when self employed; where I am free to move and grow without restrictions.

I have observed many people staying in careers and jobs that have far exceeded their 'best used by' date and often it is out of fear. I often wish they could look back on their whole life from a reverse perspective and see that it is only diminishing you to stay in anything that is not lighting you up, and that there is always something better out there. Like I said though, the leap of faith approach isn't for all and as a Career Consultant I learned how to help people step their way safely out of the old and into the new. Learning how to help people remove those self imposed barriers led me onto the path where I am today, so there seems to be quite a Divine plan to it all.

It is never too late to move into a new career or even start your first career, as my daughter, Jessica proved recently. She left school without any qualifications, had a child at a very young age but since then, has rediscovered a love for learning. Through self directed learning at a correspondence school, she passed two years worth of secondary education in only one year, flying through her study, at the same time bringing up a toddler. This accelerated learning compared to her negative response to school, was like night and day. She has since moved into an apprenticeship in a male dominated industry and is at the top of her training. She did this all by herself, once she found the motivation and confidence within herself. For this, I am very proud of her as she had many hurdles to leap to get there.

Good planning with intuitive knowing, combined with a good dose of synchronicity landing opportunities in our laps, is what we all hope for when embarking on our next career choice. Louise Hay, publishing her first book at age sixty, firstly having to set up her own publishing company to do so, is an inspiration to me that it is never too late or too difficult to fulfil your dreams.

Message: Career or Calling

What is it that pulls us to our chosen career or calling? Is it chance or design? When we find ourselves in a particular job or career we would be wise to stop and ask ourselves, does this enhance our life in some way, enrich our Being? Regardless of what particular job we are currently in, we can ask ourselves this question. Are we there by choice or by necessity? What is it in this particular career or job that is drawing us to it?

Throughout our life we fulfil many jobs for many purposes and it is how we feel when we are within that space that is more important than what we are actually doing. We could have the best job in the world and still not be happy, depending on how we feel within ourselves. We could have the most menial of jobs and feel joyous. In order to move from career to calling we must first be able to identify how we are within the current space that we occupy. Does it feel expansive and energised to be in this space or do we feel reduced and minimized? We can change how we feel about our current situation and from this position of growth and expansion, this then allows us to move into an even more enhanced position.

As we move through life, we have many choices in front of us, one of which is how we are going to make our way in life. The motivator of earning a living can lead us into either a career or a calling. There is a subtle difference between career and calling. A career is something that we choose consciously which could be determined by our family background, what our peers are doing, what's available in our environment at that time. A calling is something quite different.

A calling is when we are energetically pulled towards something that enhances our Being at every level. When we have a calling, there is nothing, there is no obstacle that will get in the way of achieving or moving towards that calling. It is so strong within us and defies all logic. We just keep moving towards this calling at a level that far exceeds anything else that's called career.

Whereas a career can move through phases and change throughout different periods in our life, a calling is like that thread that runs through us for this whole lifetime, motivates us and drives us, and leads us to wherever it is we need to go. A calling will be supported at every level by the universe as this is something that has to be done and there is no deviating from that. Having free will or free won't, if this calling is ignored or defied it can create a disharmony or even disease in our energetic being, to the point that we are not able to rest, or be well with ourselves without this calling. In some lifetimes this calling is too strong to be ignored, and if we do it is at our own peril.

Why is it that some people have this calling and others don't?

Given that this lifetime is not isolated and it is part of a complete journey, just one step in that complete journey, when we have a calling in this lifetime it overrides all else in our life and becomes the pivotal step, like that shining star that we just have to follow. It can be very hard for the people around them, and their loved ones, to understand why this calling is so strong. The risk of living this lifetime with a calling, is that we may not achieve the balance that we need to also live this human life, understanding that we also have a life outside our calling. This is a great challenge for those people who have that calling.

The great challenge is not to see it as a conflict between your calling and other parts of your life but as a way of balancing out that which we need to do spiritually for ourselves, for our actual soul being, and that which we need to do for our human self, without dividing or separating them. There can be no division or separation as that is when the disharmony and disease begin. We need to understand that this calling and our human experience can move alongside each other fluidly and easily, with one supporting the other. That is the way of our Being this lifetime.

So whether you have a career or a calling this lifetime, whichever it is, it's perfect for you at this time. To do anything other than accept and embrace that is to bring struggle and pain into your life. It is a truly wonderous thing to have that calling in this lifetime, and it is a channelled use of energy to achieve great things for your Self and other people and humanity. Also for those around the person with the calling, to be alongside them on this journey is also an honour.

Meditation: Career or Calling

Once again, bring your attention to the breath as it rises and it falls. Bring your attention to the area around the heart as the breath rises and as it falls, and bringing into that area of the heart, a colour to support this meditation. Any colour that you choose or any colour that you are given, it is one and the same. Bring into that heart centre your current situation, whether it be career or calling, letting it rest and reside within that heart centre.

Regardless of whether this current situation brings you joy or pain, bring it into that heart centre and allow it to rest and reside in that area for either transformation or integration into our Being. Allowing this current situation to be bathed in that beautiful colour, and to be transformed and released, or transformed and integrated. This allows you to get some more understanding and learning from this current situation, whether that be to learn to accept and grow with this current situation, or whether it be to release it.

Understand that this current situation is a reflection of aspects of your Being. It is perfect, at this point in time, for whatever your Being needs to have taken from it. Allow this current situation, bathed in that colour to float out and through your Being. Allow it to move gently throughout your body, throughout your energy field, bathed in that beautiful colour. Understand that by having this current situation transformed, to whatever it needs to be transformed to, will allow you either to accept and grow from it, or to accept and release it joyfully. If your current situation is that you don't have any current career or calling, that also is perfect because into this state of Being will come a sense of acceptance, and allowance. Allow whatever needs to happen to happen, to bring to you whatever it is that you so desire. Also, understand that this career or calling is just one aspect of you, that there are many aspects of you that are all integrated.

Whatever is happening right now is perfect for you. You need to find that acceptance and joy within that, before moving to wherever it is you need to move to. With this floating through you and around you, moving up into your head and down through your body, and radiating out around your Being, bringing you into harmony. Whatever it is you have, or are about to have, there are multitudes of different careers and callings that may take you through this pathway, this lifetime, and that's ok too.

So from this position, whether that be uncertainty in your life regarding this career or calling or whether there be absolute certainty, know that this is perfect for you at this time. From this state of Being, allow into your life whatever is meant to come through. Enjoy this blissful state of being in the present moment. When you're ready, knowing that this will continue, gently come back into your body, into your heart centre, containing all that needs to be contained in that heart centre, that connects you out to the whole at any time you choose. Gently open your eyes when you're ready.

Chapter 5
Abundance

Happiness resides not in possessions and not in gold,
the feeling of happiness dwells in the soul.

–Democritus

My Human Experience

I find the topic of abundance a fascinating one and it comes up a lot with clients and in workshops. It is so subjective, and people get really caught up in scarcity not realising that in doing so it just brings in more of the same. Easy for you, some may say!

Growing up I had many mixed messages about abundance as I observed Mum soldiering on as a full time working single Mum; reliably bringing in her modest income from teaching while Dad skylarked around with his music, being a drummer in a band, juggling different self employed enterprises that seemed to work at times but didn't seem to last. Although growing up pretty poor, I am glad as it taught me to appreciate the things I had earned or was given.

Luckily also, I must have seen how Dad's life was much more fun and I have never tied myself down or limited my freedom just in order to have security. This trusting that I will always be okay, rather than living in fear, has meant I have taken some pretty crazy gambles on things such as buying unpredictable real estate, or leaving well paid professions to take off and go travelling. I don't think I've ever regretted one of these choices though and I always seem to have abundance around me. By abundance, I mean I have never had to go hungry or had nowhere to sleep.

Of course, it is a state of mind as abundance to me is being alive to experience all that is around us. As long as I'm around nature or animals I feel truly abundant, which is why I decided to put the nature reading and meditation in this chapter.

So often people get caught up in the minutiae of dollars and cents and although, of course, it is important to balance your books, pay your mortgage, do your returns etc, if it's occupying too much of your thoughts, that you don't have enough, whether it be money, love, clothes, etc etc, then it will just keep bringing you more of the same. I guess it's that old gratitude rule again, that if you look around you in appreciation and gratitude, it brings in more. I still do this sometimes at the end of the day. I think of three things I have been grateful for that day and when I wake up, I think of three things I am looking forward to. This simple exercise has helped keep me in a state of abundance, although of course when things go pear shaped, as they sometimes do, funnily the first thing to go out the window is this, when it should be the most important thing to do.

As I said before, abundance is such a state of mind and when I've travelled to very poor countries and seen the sense of community and caring, as people sit around the table sharing simple food, it is truly abundant and a reminder to question, actually how much do we really need?

I've observed some patterns around money with both myself and others, such as when money comes our way, we quickly spend it or go back into debt. Growing up poor meant subconsciously I was more comfortable with this as it was familiar. This perpetual merry go round of the wealth and poverty cycle was exhausting. When I finally got off that and realised I could be comfortable and at peace with or without money it flowed to me a lot easier and I kept it.

Keeping abundance in the flow is something I've also had to learn. Spending it is actually important to keep the abundance flowing and rather than deplete the resources, it in fact brings more back around in the flow cycle. Not just money of course, but gifts of time, resources and talents. When we give out, we receive as well. Receiving is so important and again, we are often taught it is selfish but in fact receiving with gratitude benefits all parties.

When I was little, I was incredibly lucky and used to win all sorts of things. My sister said I was so tinny I would rust. That happy optimism seemed to work well for me and it was a natural part of me without me thinking it was a big deal. I don't bother buying lotto as I feel content with how things are in my life and maybe someone else would benefit more from it than me. Never having had a reliable partner, being self sufficient has been my normal state of being and I can't imagine having to rely on someone else for my security. I love being in charge of my own life and find that quite empowering. That doesn't mean to say I don't enjoy being taken out and treated of course.

I've noticed people almost put their life and happiness on hold until the big break. I'm not sure what they're waiting for or how they think it will change their life but being grateful for those things you already have is a fantastic place to start the abundance flowing. It's a bit of a paradox of course, as you become happier with what you have so you're comfortable with or without whatever you previously thought you needed to have. I think it's all part of the great cosmic joke.

I've noticed some people use money and objects as a kind of payoff for feeling guilty about not being there for their loved ones. It really is a poor replacement and leads to distorted values. The gift of time is one that really counts and being present for that person. When I had my grandson to play, all he wanted was for me to sit with him and be part of his play, endlessly running his toy cars around his car mat. Such a simple game but it gave him total pleasure to have my undivided attention. I think back to when my children were small and I know I didn't do this as much as I could have, being more preoccupied with getting those jobs done and having a tidy house. Hindsight is really not much use, apart from realising I can do it differently now.

As a kid, when we were all going through the emotional turmoil of my father having left, my escape was to go into the native bush around our house with my brother and sister. We would spend all day in there exploring, swinging off the vines, building huts, making dams in the stream and other exciting activities that kids love to do. As we got older, we seemed to drift apart and seek out our own form of entertainment. Mine was riding horses at our local farmer's place and that became my escape from the tedium of chores at home and family dramas. This love of animals, in particular horses, gave me an outlet to express myself and I'm not sure how I would have coped without that. It seemed to give me a resilience and determination that stayed with me.

We all saved frantically at great insistence from me and my first pony was a stubborn, ex riding school horse, so she knew all the tricks. Me, being a total novice, would be subjected to all sorts of bad behaviour from her. My mother found this an endless form of entertainment as I would arrive home, berating the horse for all the bad behaviours my mother complained of in me! What a mirror for me to have, not that I appreciated it at the time. Understanding now, that all the people, animals, and situations in our life are mirrors for us to look at aspects of ourselves, it was my first experience of this, not to be ignored. It's a bit hard to blame others when you realise they are just reflecting something about yourself.

From these early experiences, I never felt like I lacked anything even though we had little spare money. Being out in nature fed me on so many levels, in so many ways that a television or play station game couldn't have. Even now, if I start to feel depleted in any way, I take myself off into nature and suddenly it all seems ok again. I'm sure most people are like that, maybe not realising though, how big a part nature has to play in our lives.

Message: Connecting with Nature

Nature is all around us. We're immersed in Nature. It's within us. We are connected to it on many levels. Nature is part of our intrinsic being. Nature is all that is natural around us and within us. To connect with nature is to reconnect with ourselves at a far deeper level than we are conscious of. When we become one with Nature we become one with our Self and we are whole and complete.

Nature is perfection personified without any effort or striving. Whatever happens within nature is perfect, as it follows in a cycle of life and death, growth and regeneration. It's ever circulating as are we. When we connect with nature either externally or internally we connect at a level which far exceeds what our human mind can perceive. At a cellular level we resonate in a way that we can never achieve with our minds.

Nature is our teacher. Are we ready to listen to the lessons of Nature?

What are those lessons?

As we tune in with Nature we learn much about ourselves. We learn to experience what expands us and helps us grow and we learn to recognise that which shuts us down and isn't in our best interests. We learn to recognise what inhibits our growth. Just like the flower and the plant move towards the light, so too do we become familiar with what brings us towards the light.

As we allow ourselves to move towards the light, that allows for our growth, so simple. The flower and the plant don't have to think about it. They lean towards that light and bask in that warmth and that glow of that energy of the light.

How to connect with nature?

Nature is all around us. It's in the wind that is touching our skin. It's in the feel of things, the feel of the grass under our feet, or water as we swim in the ocean. Even the salt that we taste when we swim in the ocean or even stand in the ocean breeze and taste that salt. It's in the vivid colours that we see, the vivid blue sky or the dark deep grey of the clouds. The many nuances of green that we see in the trees and the plants, not to mention all the amazing rainbow of colours of the flowers. All around us is nature to be experienced through our senses.

As we allow ourselves to absorb nature and be absorbed into nature on many levels, we can expand our essence and grow and become one with nature until there is no distinction between Self and nature. We are nature and nature is us.

As with all things that are living in nature we move towards that which expands us, not what constricts us. The more we immerse ourselves with nature, the more we learn to recognise that which, in our life, expands our being, and that which in our life constricts us. If we can recognise this distinction, we can choose to go towards that which expands us and brings us to that light. Then our choices and our decision-making in life becomes very simple. All we have to do is go within and experience whether we're expanded or constricted within ourselves. Whether we're growing or we're diminishing. The more we move towards that which grows us and expands us, the more we grow, the more abundance we get. Conversely, the more we choose to go with the experience which constricts us and diminishes us, the more we become diminished and our world becomes diminished and smaller.

If we choose to live in a world of growth and expansion then we have ultimate, unlimited possibilities given to us. Nature provides us with everything that we need and we are nature so therefore we have everything within us that we need. We need look no further than within, once we are connected with nature.

To experience this with nature we will do a short meditation that you can do at anytime in the presence of nature which, of course, is all the time.

Meditation: Connecting with Nature

Close your eyes, and once again bring your attention to your breathing. Notice the natural rise and fall, just as we notice that ebb and flow of the tide and the waves. If you're fortunate to be outside or surrounded by nature, notice any sounds, scents or feelings on your skin, of nature, or the touch of nature around you. If you're not in direct contact with nature, just call that in. Call in that experience or a time when you've been in touch with nature. It may be the wind, it may be the water, it may be the warmth of the sun on your skin, on your face, or the feel of the rain on your skin. It could be the sounds of the leaves in the tree or the sounds of water rushing by in a river, or that pulsing sensation of the water in the waves, or even the trickle of a stream. Connecting to a sensation through our five senses, or one of our five senses, to an aspect of nature, allows your Self to connect with this.

As your breathing in your heart centre expands and energises through the breath in the heart centre, and connecting this heart centre with the sensation of nature, allow that sensation to become part of your breath, part of your heart centre.

As you are now a part of nature, so is nature a part of you, and allow this expansion of nature within your heart centre to extend out beyond your body, beyond your energy field, until it becomes all of nature and nature becomes all of you.

Enjoy this connection, knowing that you have this at any time and at all times by opening your heart centre and reaching, extending out and drawing in, all at the same time. Knowing that this is now part of your being, when you're ready, gently open your eyes and come back into the room.

Chapter 6

Connecting With Others

The supreme happiness in life is the conviction that we are loved—loved for ourselves, or rather, loved in spite of ourselves.

–Victor Hugo

My Human Experience

As with many people, I have had both profoundly wonderful experiences and also profoundly painful experiences in my connections with others. As a child, as with many children, I was an open book and able to connect with others easily and effortlessly. Yet, as life proceeded to do what it does with family dynamics, school systems, peer pressure etc, I gradually shrunk back within myself to a much safer place of Being. There is the hurt child within many of us and it is this that really needs the healing before any other changes can take place.

How we connect on so many levels is very intriguing. As with many others, the times I have been thinking of someone and they phone or email at about the same time, leads me to realise that we connect not just on the physical level but on the energetic level as well. Within the field of New Biology, perceptions are changing. Our thoughts are increasingly viewed as energy. It's energy, just at

55

another frequency, so it makes total sense that we connect through our thoughts. This is a very humbling realisation when you think how often we have negative thoughts about someone or something.

I also used to think that the encounters we had on a daily basis were random, chance, whatever you like to call it. But again I have come to realise that there is no such thing as a chance encounter, and that every interaction we have is purposeful and leaves an energetic footprint. It makes you very mindful of the interactions we have. Another favourite book of mine by Mitch Albom,'s, *The Five People You Meet in Heaven*, helped change my thinking very early on in my journey.

I also then started to notice the difference it made with others depending on my attitude. It is very sobering when I think back over some of my past encounters, but at least the awareness is there now. The comment from my daughter after she read this book made me realise she was having similar thoughts as well. Gulp! The realisation that every encounter we have, has a consequence. It makes you very mindful of how you treat others.

Over the course of my spiritual journey, I have come into contact many times with the readings on the Lemurian culture and have always felt a strong affiliation with them. When I started working with the PSYCH-K process as an Instructor, I was delighted to discover that the PSYCH-K spiritual retreats which I now facilitate, are in fact based on the Lemurian Law of One, in that we are all connected to each other and everything. Their culture is an ancient one, when the need for spoken words was unnecessary, and their connection to nature and energy was all intertwined as part of their Being. At a recent retreat we had on the small island of Lembongan, close to Bali, we discovered through a series of synchronicities, a location in Lavinia Beach that had a Temple of One with a similar philosphy. After our retreat a few of us continued on to visit this Temple and the Lemurian energy vortex located there. Staying with the resident Buddhist priest and experiencing the magic of this place and the people, was one of those special moments. It was the feeling of being in exactly the right place, right time with the right people.

My connection with others has not always been so harmonious and it has been one of my harder lessons in life, to be part of a whole. Being on my own has been the easy part for me, and the challenge is being in the presence of others and feeling comfortable, safe and connected. In the past I would often be on the defensive which made for poor communication and connection. Always preferring to have a small group of friends to interact with, rather than be a social butterfly. Studying Carl Jung's personality type went some way in gaining an understanding of why this was and how to achieve the balance in my interactions.

Since being back on my spiritual path, it has been noticeably easy to be around others and feel connected in a comfortable, easy way without having to prove anything to myself and others.

Message: Connecting With Others

Connecting with others in our daily encounters can present challenges and potential for both joy and discomfort. When we encounter another Being that resonates with us at either the same vibration frequency or a different vibration frequency, it can present one of two challenges for us.

If there is something in the other person that we recognise in ourselves, that we are not comfortable with and are not yet ready to face, it can bring to the surface feelings and responses that do not sit with us comfortably. As we are not yet ready to face this within ourselves, when we see it in others it brings up a myriad of emotions and responses that make us uncomfortable. In response to this discomfort, what we may not be ready to face yet, we will often seek to displace onto the other person. This again can present itself in several ways.

We may make a judgement about them, a criticism which in some way shifts the attention to the other person, when in fact it is something within our Self that we are really making the judgement about. We may also attempt to create a situation where the other person is at fault when, again, it is our Self we are trying to direct the attention away from. Why does this come about? Why is there such conflict within the world, at a level both of individuals and of nations?

Again, it is a reluctance to directly face that within our Self which we are not quite ready to face.

Imagine that when we interact, throughout our day, with the shop keeper, our colleagues, or our family, we are actually interacting with an aspect of our Self. It may be an interaction that we enjoy embracing, or that we feel discomfort with because it is an aspect we are not ready to accept within ourselves.

How can we change these interactions with both individual beings and collective groups, to be encounters of joyful recognition and abundant experiences?

Simply by opening our heart to the possibility that all these encounters are in fact opportunities to re-acquaint ourselves with yet another aspect of our Self, to recognise it and embrace it, is to accept it unconditionally. When we do this we have released all judgement, and criticism. Thus we release judgement about our Self, as well, in doing so.

As we take each encounter throughout the day, and store these experiences in our Being as positive and interesting aspects of our Self, we open up the space to move on to more positive and interesting encounters, rather than staying focussed on such limiting encounters and experiences.

Many of us recognise that we keep calling up the same experiences over and over again and may wonder why this is so. Until we fully embrace and accept that these experiences are not about anyone else except our Self, they will keep repeating. They will not repeat once we have accepted them as our own.

Meditation: Connecting With Others

To release any interactions of this nature that are creating discomfort, close your eyes and bring your attention to your breathing. Notice the rise and fall of the breath in the chest area. Allow the breathing to fill that area of your heart centre, expanding and energising it as you do so. As you stay in your heart centre with your breath, bring into it an experience of a time with someone or something where your reaction was anything less than happiness. As you think about this interaction or experience, bring it into your heart centre and create the shape of a heart around this picture or feeling. As you continue to fill this area with your breath allow it now to bring in a colour. Bathe this experience in that colour that you chose. Stay with this breath as you fill that heart and the experience with that beautiful colour, bathing the experience in light to fill your Being. As you fill this area with light, notice how the feelings that were once feelings of discomfort are fading and there is a feeling of connectedness and understanding. This experience, being an expression of your Self, is now filled with love and understanding.

As we integrate this feeling of love and understanding into our Being we realise that this is in fact a gift of recognition for our Self to remember and restore to a place of acceptance. Taking a copy of this beautiful heart with all its knowledge and happiness, take it up through a rainbow of light to your head and when the copy of the heart is up in your head click it into place. Click!

Knowing that this new understanding is now part of yourself, to reconnect all aspects of yourself, gently open your eyes and come back into the room when you are ready.

Chapter 7
Love and Healing

"Love is the great miracle cure. Loving ourselves works miracles in our lives."

–Louise Hay

My Human Experience

As I ponder on this final chapter, I at first see the titles as separate issues to be addressed then realise that of course one must intrinsically go with the other. When we allow love into our life, for our Self and others, the healing is automatic.

The titles were not chosen by me consciously as they came in with the rest of the intuitive download I received in the early hours of the Wesak Moon, so it finally dawns on me that this too is an area in my own life I need to address and acknowledge, as I have had to in all the previous chapters.

As with many people, within me is the hurt child, friend, wife, mother, work colleague, all in need of love and healing. I reminisce back to that outgoing, happy child I was and see how life's experiences and hurts slowly dimmed that light Being down to become guarded and defensive, and I mourn for that happy child.

I see it also in the people around me, my loved ones and clients and I feel for them also. At the same time I celebrate in the joy of the journey back to who we really are. How exquisite is that journey of enlightenment and it is to be savoured and enjoyed. How to bring that happiness back into all our lives has not been something I have consciously sought, I realise as I sit typing these words, but something that has driven me for years to seek, as I know so many others do.

I reflect on my layers of defence, and those of others, whether that is to shut down emotionally, or use substances and behaviours that numb or distract us, add layers of padding to the body to protect ourselves, or whatever it takes to feel safe. It all makes total sense to me that we do these things to mask the hurt, but I also know that there is a way to regain that joy and happiness.

My niece once asked me how she could keep her little girl safe from life. Even to have to ask such a question is sobering in the enormity of it. My reply was to let her daughter respond and do what intuitively she knows is right for herself, rather than what our social politeness expects of us, thus shutting down her own sense of what she needs and what is safe for her. Let her decide who she wants to give a hug to rather than doing it on demand to gratify others.

My healing journey has been a long one and it is still continuing but the more I learn to love and accept myself, the more my relationships and my life heals and improves. It just keeps getting better and easier and I celebrate in the gratitude of finally being able to get out of my own way.

What a paradox life is and a great cosmic joke really. That we all try so hard when really all we need to do is get out of our own mind and trust and allow. It sounds so simple and I have seen it play out time and time again in my own life and those of my loved ones and clients when they finally see it too. We have some great laughs about ourselves in this regard when we finally get around an issue we have been doing battle with, trying to fix, and then finding the solution right under our nose.

The more I get out of my own way, life brings in more and more synchronicities and gifts. Surrender sounds like a big leap into the abyss but the times I have fully done this, and jumped through the fear barrier, there has only ever been a better outcome in the big picture. I watch the struggles we have as humans and reflect that it is not my job to fix other people's lives, only my own, and in doing so, only then am

I able to be there for others. Again, a paradox, but it makes sense on reflection. I have to remind myself often of this, as I see my children struggle through with their lives, making many of the same mistakes I made and their father made, but knowing that they are so much more than their early childhood programming. I look forward to the time when the realisation dawns for them, as they release what is not of them, and they can once again be those amazing, beautiful creatures they were and, of course, still are.

The other aspect of our healing journey is allowing the greater part or spiritual aspects of the Universe into our daily lives. Experiences into the spiritual realms have been a haphazard process with me over the years and I have given myself a huge fright at times when I have ventured into territories and realms that I wasn't quite ready for.

This channelling of my Higher Self has felt the safest and most comfortable part of all my journeying. Like many people and most animals, I am sensitive to the spiritual realms. I have had a few experiences with spirits, just passed over, whilst being around their loved ones. I can only equate it to a feeling of instinctive, intuitive awareness with skin and hair reacting to the presence of another level of being.

At the time, not understanding what it was, fear was my automatic response. After this happening a few times, and finding out from that person that a loved one had just passed, it made sense that my intuition had been alerted on another level that their presence was there. Visits to clairvoyants over the years, with mostly accurate reports of my loved ones passing and details of my current life, have made me comfortable with the understanding that we are spiritual beings having a human experience. More recently, I have started seeing images of people around that are not of this world, but Beings on another energetic level and surprisingly it has not been at all disconcerting so maybe I am ready for the next level of awareness.

The surrogation healing work that I do with others, communicates across all levels of Being, this lifetime and other lifetimes so it makes sense that the connection doesn't stop when we die. Energy is all around us and when I have felt the different levels of energy from Spirit it has taken a while to be comfortable with it.

Years ago I bought an American Indian mandela which had a very powerful energy and I had it in my room while I slept. That night I woke in a living nightmare, screaming and incoherent having tapped into something that was too strong for me to handle. On fully awakening I had lost several years of memories so I have a great respect for the power of Spirit and I am very careful who and what I have around me now.

I have found the same with crystals as they also magnify energy and I am aware of being mindful with them, cleansing them and being careful where they are placed. Being grounded and protected is a vital step when exploring other energy forms. I have only had a glimpse into these realms and look forward to expanding my awareness as I grow in my journey. For over ten years I kept away from all this type of work as a reaction to the fear of the power of these forces, but am only now tipping my toes back in the water, as I am more grounded and mature. Being in nature has been the strongest connection point for me, and it is in the presence of nature that I am able to truly open up and allow.

Recently, while walking in the Australian bush I was taking a photo on my phone of an amazing tree that had its roots wrapped around a huge boulder. After taking the photo, an image of an aborigine with blue feathered loin cloth came into my side vision, silently requesting my respect for the bush and its ancestors by not taking photos. He was not threatening but was very clear in his intention. It was sobering and reminded me that we inhabit this earth with many other Beings. Being mindful of that, is part of our journey. From this encounter, once again, I felt very connected to the realisation that everything and everyone is part of a whole.

These are baby steps that I have taken and I'm not sure where it will lead. While I stay open and curious, anything is possible. In learning to love and accept myself, I have noticed that I am then able to give and receive love more easily than I imagined possible. I often ask myself, could it be this easy? The results speak for themselves and I am learning to trust more in this as my life journey becomes more enriched and abundant.

Message: Healing Our Mind & Emotions

If we look at our heart and our head, they're connected. Our head, encompassing the mind and the brain, are where they're interconnecting. Yet they've found that people, in fact, can have very little left of their brain and still function, as the mind is still operating.

Where do these thoughts come from? Why is our mind so active? Our mind is where most people are having the problems in their life, the thoughts and feelings that are going around and around in their minds. If these thoughts and these feelings arise from emotional responses to our experiences and our emotions are in our heart, then it would make sense that the healing needs to be done at the heart level. Our emotional hurts in our heart manifest and arise as thoughts and feelings and attitudes to all these experiences that we've had, and had emotional responses and reactions to.

When we heal our heart, these thoughts and feelings that we no longer wish to have running in our mind, dissipate and dissolve. When we heal at the heart level, balance is restored in mind, body and spirit. In healing our heart, from that hurt, all other hurt heals, whether it be illness of the mind or illness of the body, dis-ease of the mind, dis-ease of the body. These are external manifestations of internal hurt. That hurt of the Inner Self.

With heart healing we can once again become heart happiness, as that automatically creates happiness in our mind, our body and our spirit. Happiness at all levels of being, not just at a cellular level but happiness right out and far reaching, out to everything and everyone.

Meditation: Healing Our Mind & Emotions

To create this heart healing we bring our attention once again to our breath. Close your eyes if you wish. Focus on that rise and fall of the breath, the breath being the life force energy. Bring the breath into the heart centre and fill the heart centre with light. Create a heart shape and you may choose any colour to fill that heart. Expand that breath from that heart, so the colour that you chose, spreads out around your body. As it does, send all that healing and happiness throughout every cell in your body, and in every energy wave around your body, and around your Being. And filling that Being with seven deep breathes, each one healing an aspect of your body, of your mind, of your spirit, that calls for healing from your heart centre. Each of those seven breaths speaks to a different aspect of your Self and resonates at a different frequency within your Self.

The colours may change with each breath and that's perfect for what we're doing here. And as you notice that there are parts of your body beginning to activate when they have had this healing breath, allow that movement, whether it be to release something or to activate something that has long been inert or asleep.

Continue that breathe until all seven breaths of that life force are complete and your body's energy is flowing as one, free flowing and free. Know that this connection is all throughout your body. This rainbow of colour is all throughout your mind and right out, reaching out. When you're ready, gently open your eyes and come back into the room.

Message: Soul Healing

Everyone has the ability to heal themselves. They have the ability within themselves to heal whatever needs healing. To be able to heal ourselves from within and access that internal awareness we need to become aware. We need to become the watcher and the observer of what is happening within us rather than looking externally through assistance and help.

Often what we have is directly within us, if we take that time to be still and go within, to actually find out what is happening within us at any given time in that moment. As our reactions, responses, emotions and feelings surface as signals, that is the critical point to go within, become aware and check to see what is happening within us rather than externalising our reaction or response to somebody or something as being the cause.

As we go within ourselves, notice, and bring our attention to our internal response and become aware, stay neutral around that, and you may have a response like 'That's interesting. I didn't know that. I didn't know that about myself'.

When we take our attention within, rather than allowing it to expand out to the causal event, then we take ownership. We're in control of our own lives rather than allowing external events, people and situations to determine our happiness. It is also an opportunity at this point to realize that what is happening may be a response to something that has happened earlier and this is a chance to heal old wounds. When we heal old wounds, we then cease to respond and react in old ways. These external events and situations just slip past us without having that heavy impact on our system and causing that emotional and physiological response that sometimes can make us uncomfortable.

These responses can also bring us joy and that's interesting too. But if there is healing to be done then we go within and give our attention to what is happening, as the observer. Then we can discontinue old negative patterns from continuing in our future life. At any given point as life and people bring these situations into our life they're actually gifts and opportunities for us to address what may be old responses.

As we observe our own responses and behaviour objectively, it allows us to grow and become aware. Then awareness and growth happen simultaneously and effortlessly without having to work hard at it to break old patterns. All we have to do is become aware of what is actually happening right now, at this point in time, and that then changes everything that has been, and everything that is coming. We can create new pathways to explore in our life that previously may have been unavailable to us because of old responses to old behaviours.

It's a truly wondrous thing that we can set ourselves free, and that we need to look no further than ourselves to do so. We have all the answers within us, and then when we no longer respond in the old ways, we become that shining light for others to see what is within them. This allows others to take ownership of what is happening in their lives. We need do nothing to help the people and our loved ones around us, other than looking within ourselves. In doing that we then allow the space for them to look within themselves, to heal themselves, which is the most powerful form of healing on this planet.

This is why, if you observe animals in nature, when they're unwell, they will find a space to be. Their loved ones, the animals around them, will just hold that space, allowing them to be, to go within and do whatever is necessary, whether that be to heal at this point, or to pass over if they're ready.

Meditation: Soul Healing

Bringing your attention to your breath as it rises and it falls, allow it to rise and fall freely. As your breath rises and falls freely, notice and become aware of any places or spaces in your body or in your mind or even in your spirit where this breath is not freely moving. As you bring your attention and awareness to these areas that are unavailable to this life force energy, notice that they start to tingle and awaken. In receiving this life force energy, the breath, the tingling starts to dissolve and as it dissolves, this area in your body or your mind or your spirit begins to integrate into your whole system.

Allow this breath to flow throughout your body. There is no beginning and no end to that flow. That flow just is, ever moving like the rise and fall of our breath, just as the waves rise and fall, as we allow that to flow smoothly through our body, clearing away all blockages and resistance. We allow all things to flow smoothly within us and around us, experiencing that peaceful, settled state.

Knowing that any time we feel any resistance, whether it be mental, emotional, physical or spiritual, by bringing our attention to that area, or to that space, and energising it with the life force breathe, we can aid in releasing that resistance.

This is our gift to our Self that we have at any time, any place, any dimension of Being. Being assured of this, when you are ready, bring that breath and attention back to your heart centre, slow that down and gently coming back to the room, opening your eyes when you're ready.

Conclusion

$\mathcal{H}$aving received these messages, meditations and guidance, have I achieved Heart Happiness in my life?

Still not fully but I am finding the more time I put aside to meditate and connect to myself, the easier it is to stay in that space while living my everyday human life. The challenges that once would have sent me into a downward spiral, now skim over me without having too strong an emotional reaction and effect. I am able to stay more fully present in myself, notice my responses and choose how I want to be in that present moment in time. Being centred in my heart has helped me maintain that sense of emotional balance and thus freedom from the resulting thoughts. It feels empowering to live my life this way.

As life presents repeated situations, patterns and experiences, I am becoming more aware that the Heart Happiness messages received are directly relating to what is happening at that point. When I get honest with myself, what is going on is something in me that needs to be addressed. I can then go to the relevant message and do the healing meditation. Once I acknowledge this and take action, it has been fascinating to see how quickly the energy of the experience dissipates and shifts.

Not knowing what the future may bring, I can only stay fully present here and now, expanding to my full potential at each moment in time and allowing myself to become whatever I need to be.

Thank you for sharing my journey and I sincerely hope it helps you in some way, with your own journey.

Julienne Rose

69

Summary of Meditations

1. Establishing a Heart Connection

2. Aligning Heart & Mind

3. Clearing Unwanted Thoughts Healing

4. Relationships

5. Clearing Energy Blockages in the Body/Mind/Spirit.

6. Affirmations & Beliefs

7. Receiving Messages from your Higher Self

1. Establishing a Heart Connection

To establish a heart connection is to be free of your mind, free of the limitations of thought. With practice you will be able to stay connected to your heart, thus accessing the heart intelligence at all times.

- ♥ With eyes opened or closed, bring your attention to your breathing.
- ♥ Focus your breathing into your heart centre around the chest area and expand and energise that area.
- ♥ Know that this heart centre is the channel to your Higher Self.
- ♥ When in connection with your heart centre, your mind is still and at peace.
- ♥ If you choose to, allow a colour to fill your heart centre.
- ♥ This colour may be used to enhance and heal whatever needs to be healed.
- ♥ Know that at any time you focus your breath into your heart centre you are connected to your highest state of Being.
- ♥ The more you practice this, the more you will be free of your mind and be at peace.

2. Aligning Heart & Mind

Our subconscious mind is responsible for at least 95% of what runs our life. As this is often a summation of our life experiences and beliefs, it is useful to integrate the heart intelligence to ensure our mind is operating at optimum efficiency and clarity.

- ♥ With your eyes open or closed, bring your attention to your breathing.
- ♥ Focus your breathing into your heart centre around the chest area and expand and energise that area.
- ♥ Imagine a heart shape in any colour that you choose.
- ♥ Within this heart, gently place a picture of what it is you desire. Eg: a goal, relationship, feeling.
- ♥ Create a rainbow and connect this from your heart to your head.
- ♥ Send a copy of the coloured heart with the picture in it, up to your head.
- ♥ As you see the two hearts connected by the rainbow, click the heart in place. **Click!**
- ♥ Knowing that this connection is in place, gently open your eyes and come back into the room.

3. Clearing Unwanted Thoughts & Feelings

We often identify with our thoughts and feelings. Whatever those thoughts and feelings are, we think we are. Yet we are so much more. In realising this, we get to choose the quality of our thoughts and feelings, thus our life.

- ♥ With eyes opened or closed, bring your attention to your breathing.
- ♥ Focus your breathing into your heart centre, the chest area and expand and energise that area.
- ♥ As a thought comes into your mind, take it down through a rainbow of coloured light for cleansing and purifying.
- ♥ Encompass that thought in your heart centre and bathe it in a colour. This can also be done with a feeling.
- ♥ That thought has now been transformed into whatever it needs to be for your highest goal.
- ♥ Knowing that you can do this at any time with any thought, gently open your eyes.

4. Healing Relationships

♥   With eyes opened or closed, bring your attention to your breathing.
♥   Focus your breathing into your heart centre around the chest area and expand and energise that area.
♥   Create a heart image in your heart centre. Fill it with a colour that you choose, or that you feel is needed for this relationship.
♥   Gently place a picture of that person or people into that heart image, encompassing it with the warmth and beauty of the colour that you have chosen.
♥   Once that heart is encompassing that relationship, extend a rainbow from the heart in your heart centre up to your head.
♥   Take a copy of that heart image with that relationship in it, up to your head and click it into place. **Click!**
♥   Know that this is safely in place, and you can recall that picture at any time and bring warmth, healing and happiness to you.

5. Clearing Energy Blockages in the Body/Mind/Spirit

This is a chance to heal old wounds at all levels and once healed we then cease to respond and react in old ways, discontinuing these patterns in our future life also. At any given point, life situations are actually gifts and opportunities for us to address what may be old hurts and responses.

♥ With eyes opened or closed, bring your attention to your breathing.

♥ Focus your breathing into your heart centre around the chest area and expand and energise that area.

♥ Notice and become aware of any places or spaces in your body, mind or spirit where this breath is not freely moving.

♥ As you bring your awareness and the breath to that area, it starts to tingle and awaken its awareness.

♥ In receiving this life force energy, the breath, it starts to dissolve this area in your body, mind or spirit and it begins to integrate into your whole system. You may allow in a healing colour to support this.

♥ Allow the breath to flow that colour smoothly throughout your body, clearing away all blockages and resistance.

♥ When you are ready, bring the breath back to your heart centre, gently opening your eyes when you're ready.

6. Affirmations & Beliefs

From the experiences we have, we receive messages about our Self, other people and the world. If the experiences are positive then we establish positive beliefs. If the experiences are negative, we establish negative beliefs. These beliefs are stored in our subconscious mind and our reality is shaped by these beliefs. To manifest our conscious goals, we need to align our subconscious beliefs with these.

- ♥ Establish a heart connection with eyes open or closed
- ♥ Place the affirmation or belief into the heart centre
- ♥ Invite or allow in a colour to support this
- ♥ Energise the heart centre with 3 deep breaths
- ♥ Run a rainbow of coloured light up to your head, from your heart
- ♥ Take a copy of this heart shape up through the rainbow to your head
- ♥ Click it into place. **Click!**

Affirmations & Beliefs To Check

- ♥ I can
- ♥ I deeply love, appreciate and accept myself
- ♥ I live in a friendly, supportive Universe
- ♥ I am worthy and deserving of all that life has to offer
- ♥ I forgive myself and others
- ♥ It is safe for me to live my life fully
- ♥ I open my heart to all that is in my highest and best good
- ♥ I embrace change as a natural part of life
- ♥ I live my life with joy and compassion
- ♥ I attract abundance into my life
- ♥ All is perfect, whole and complete in my world
- ♥ I trust my choices and decisions

Create some of your own affirmations & beliefs. They must be about yourself, be positive and in the present tense. Most of all they must be important & relevant to you!

Louise Hay's affirmations are a wonderful source as well.

- ♥

- ♥

- ♥

- ♥

7. Receiving Messages from Your Higher Self

To be able to access your own inner wisdom at any time is to achieve a heart coherence that will stand you in good stead in any situation. It will provide you with information and guidance that is second to none. When we go externally for guidance, we are relying on the skills of someone else that may not be consistent with what we really need. To take the time to listen to our Higher Self is the first step in doing this for ourselves. Create space each day to be still and clear away the clutter and busyness of the mind. With practice you can be in your heart space at all times, and thereby accessing your Inner Wisdom whenever needed.

- ♥ Establish a heart connection *(as per number 1)*
- ♥ Clear unwanted thoughts and feelings *(as per number 3)*
- ♥ Stay in a heart centred space to achieve a state of allowing
- ♥ Ask your Higher Self if there is anything you need to know
- ♥ Trust the first response that comes up *(allow space)*
- ♥ Ask your Higher Self any questions you may have
- ♥ Trust the first response that comes up *(allow space)*
- ♥ Thank your Higher Self for this guidance

Resources

www.hearthappiness.org

Free audio downloads of the messages and meditations as originally received.

Heart Happiness Healing Days information.

www.juliennerose.com

Julienne Rose's coaching website

www.heartmath.org

Research on the heart/mind connection

www.pathofdzar.com.au

Meditations and channelling of the energies of Dzar uniting human and spirit

About the Author

Julienne Rose is an International Instructor in personal change as well as a Wellness Coach in private practice. Her workshops take her around Australasia, helping transform people's lives, which is something she is passionate about and dedicated to.

When Julienne discovered the art of connecting with her Higher Self, she was both excited and in awe of this new level of insight and awareness. In her desire to share this knowledge, **The Heart of Happiness** came into being. To discover more about Julienne's work, please visit her website at www.juliennerose.com and also the website dedicated to **The Heart of Happiness** with free meditation downloads at www.hearthappiness.org